THE DIETITIAN'S GUIDE TO POLYCYSTIC OVARY SYNDROME

ANGELA GRASSI

Luca Publishing
551 West Lancaster Avenue
Suite 305
Haverford, PA 19041
(484) 252-9028
www.PCOSnutrition.com

Jeff Harris, Editor

Cover design by Christine Davis

Manufactured in the United States of America

The Dietitian's Guide to Polycystic Ovary Syndrome

Written by Angela Grassi

ISBN 13: 978-0-615-15456-5

TABLE OF CONTENTS

REVIEWERS

Jeffrey E. Harris, DrPH, MPH, RD, LDN
Associate Professor of Dietetics
West Chester University of Pennsylvania
West Chester, Pennsylvania

Stephanie Mattei, Psy.D.
Adjunct Faculty
Department of Psychology
LaSalle University
Philadelphia, PA

Lynn Monahan Couch, MPH, RD, LDN
Instructor of Dietetics
West Chester University of Pennsylvania
West Chester, Pennsylvania

Jessica Setnick, MS, RD, LD
Private Practice
Dallas, Texas

Katherine D. Sherif, MD, FACP
Director, Center for Women's Health and
The Polycystic Ovary Syndrome Program
Drexel University College of Medicine
Philadelphia, Pennsylvania

ACKNOWLEDGEMENTS

I HAVE MANY PEOPLE TO thank for their support in the completion of this book. First, I want to thank Christine Davis for designing such a fantastic cover for this book. I have such admiration for your talent.

Thank you Lisa Marasco for sharing your insightful and well-written thesis showing the connection between PCOS and insufficient milk supply.

Thank you to Jessica Setnick, my soul-sister dietitian, for reviewing this book and for your support, encouragement, and friendship.

To my good friend, Dr. Stephanie Mattei: you are a lifesaver and I cannot thank you enough. Thank you for co-authoring Chapter 2, Psychological Aspects of PCOS and for reviewing this book. You are such an awesome mom and therapist. I appreciate your time, expertise, support, and friendship.

Thank you also to Michelle Shwarz for co-authoring the chapter on Psychological Aspects of PCOS and for being so dedicated to supporting women with PCOS.

To Dr. Katherine Sherif, I can't express how much admiration and respect I have for you as a friend and physician. Your kindness, compassion, and expertise are exactly what women with PCOS need. Thank you for writing Chapter 1, Understanding PCOS. The book would not be complete without it.

A special thank you to Lynn Monahan Couch for editing and reviewing this book and for co-authoring Chapter 9. I greatly appreciate all your time, effort, advice, and encouragement. It has been wonderful working with you and forming the friendship we have. I applaud your enthusiasm and passion for learning all you can about PCOS. I look forward to collaborating on future projects together.

I want to especially thank Dr. Jeff Harris for editing and reviewing this book. I cannot thank you enough for your endless support, expertise, respect, and encouragement. Never have I met a professor liked so much by both his students and colleagues. You are a wonderful dietitian, professor, and friend and I could not have written this book without you.

I would also like to thank my family and friends for all their love and support. Becky, thank you for spending your last hurrah editing my book. Most of all, thank you to the men in my life. Luca, you have been the best little boy a new mom could ask for. Thank you for listening to me read my book aloud to you for hours on end and for being a good sleeper. Finally, I want to thank Chris. I am so lucky to have you in my life. I could not have done this without your endless love. You are my everything.

INTRODUCTION

I FELT COMPELLED TO WRITE *The Dietitian's Guide to Polycystic Ovary Syndrome* (PCOS) for several reasons. The first is that PCOS is perhaps the most complex endocrine disorder and there has been much confusion surrounding its diagnosis and treatment approaches among the medical community. This has led to numerous misdiagnoses and immense frustration and anger in women who have PCOS, all of which could have been avoided with adequate knowledge of the syndrome. Furthermore, women with PCOS are at an increased risk for obesity, cardiovascular disease, diabetes, cancer, depression, infertility, and miscarriage; early intervention aimed at preventing these is crucial.

Current treatment recommendations for PCOS emphasize the importance of dietary and lifestyle modification, thus increasing the number of referrals to dietitians for nutrition management. However, many dietitians may lack the knowledge and training to recognize or effectively treat individuals with PCOS. Some dietitians have never even heard of PCOS before. This may result from the lack of clinical studies regarding diet composition and PCOS, or because the syndrome was viewed primarily as a reproductive disorder and not diagnosed as readily as it is today. Personally, I had never heard of PCOS until after I had graduated with my master's degree in nutrition and was already working as a dietitian for a year.

Another reason I wanted to write this book is because I have PCOS and like too many women, I was misdiagnosed until I was in my late 20's. In fact, when I was diagnosed with PCOS I was already familiar with the syndrome. As a dietitian, I had treated numerous women with PCOS, yet was unable to fully recognize it for myself. This led me to question: if I hadn't been able to recognize PCOS for myself when I was already familiar with it, how are other dietitians, health professionals, or even patients going to be able to recognize it?

I remember the first time I had ever heard of polycystic ovary syndrome. It was in the year 2000 and I was working as an outpatient nutritionist for an eating disorder treatment facility. Sally, my patient who had bulimia nervosa, was recently diagnosed with PCOS when I met her. Never hearing of PCOS before, I immediately began researching the syndrome only to find limited information. The information that did exist described PCOS as a reproductive disorder associated with elevated insulin and androgen levels, weight gain, and obesity. A low carbohydrate diet was recommended.

It was at that time when I first questioned whether I had PCOS. Since puberty I have been overweight even though I have always been physically active. I never had any of the other classic PCOS symptoms of excess hair growth, acne, or irregular periods, therefore, I didn't think it was possible that I could have PCOS.

After my encounter with that first patient, I started to see many other patients like her. It was also at this time that I started gaining weight after many years of my weight being stable-and it was all accumulating in my mid-section, which never happened before. I attributed the weight gain (2-3 pounds per month) to many factors: a sedentary job, decreased metabolism, birth control pills, more eating and less physical activity. Being a dietitian, I started writing down and analyzing everything that I ate. I was not eating any more than I had before and I was certainly not eating enough to produce the weight gain that I was experiencing. It didn't make sense.

I went to see my internist to get blood work done. I suggested the possibility of having PCOS. She said, however, that she could not test for it because I was on birth control pills and they would affect the results of my hormone levels. She also said that since I always had regular periods, I could not have PCOS. All my lab results came back normal. Her answer to me about the weight gain was "watch your diet." So I figured, as I had for most of my life, that my weight was my fault. I began exercising more and continued to record my food intake. After a few more months the weight gain stopped but I was never able to lose weight.

I started noticing some other things that weren't right. For instance, I craved carbohydrates a lot more, especially sweets, and I sometimes experienced hypoglycemic episodes. My first encounter with hypoglycemia was in my senior year of college when I woke up one morning dizzy and nauseous. After eating breakfast, I got extremely dizzy to the point where I could not walk straight and had to stop and rest. I went to the health center where they diagnosed me with vertigo, said I had a virus that was going around, and prescribed me antivert. The next day I got a call telling me that the results of blood work showed my glucose reading was 40 mg/dl (normal is 70-99).

I had always wondered why I experienced hypoglycemia that day and days since. I was always careful, eating frequently and including sufficient protein with my meals and snacks. My fasting blood glucose levels had always been normal, yet I would still experience hypoglycemia at times. Several months after seeing my internist, I wasn't experiencing any change in my weight and decided to see another physician.

This time, not only did I suggest PCOS to my doctor but asked to get an oral glucose tolerance test done in addition to more lab tests. When the doctor called me with the results, she said all my hormone levels were fine and that the oral glucose tolerance test showed I had hypoglycemia (I already knew that!). She suggested I follow the South Beach Diet to lose weight and manage my hypoglycemia. What I didn't realize at the time was that she never checked my fasting insulin with the glucose test. She only tested my glucose and was not thorough in checking the hormones needed to diagnose PCOS. It also appeared that my triglyceride levels, still in normal range, were much higher than they had been the last time I had them done. I decided to stop taking birth control medication to see if my weight and triglycerides would decrease. My weight did not change and I still experienced regular periods.

I continued to see more and more patients with PCOS in my private practice and was even giving presentations on it to consumers and professionals, all while having a nagging suspicious instinct in the back of my mind telling me that I do have PCOS. My husband and I were starting to think about starting a family. At the same time, Dr. Katherine Sherif, a well-known physician who specializes in PCOS and women's health, moved back to the Philadelphia area. I made an appointment to see her thinking I could market my nutrition services to her PCOS patients. I also knew that if I had PCOS she would be the one to tell me. I had to know once and for all if I had PCOS or not, especially before trying to conceive a child.

Dr. Sherif was a model for what we wish all doctors would be: kind, compassionate, brilliant, and thorough. She took a detailed medical history on me and agreed that I should be able to lose weight with all the exercise I was doing and for the amount that I was eating. I finally felt validated that it was not my fault I wasn't able to lose weight. She also examined my skin and immediately noticed signs of acanthosis nigricans (markers of elevated insulin) on the back of my neck and knuckles. Since I am fair skinned, it had been difficult to see them. Dr. Sherif agreed that I did not have the main symptoms of PCOS but that I would have to get an ultrasound done in addition to very comprehensive blood work to rule out any other possible medical conditions. It was then that I learned that a small percentage of women with PCOS get regular periods. Later that week, I went for an ultrasound. I immediately saw the classic string of white pearls around my ovaries and it was then that I knew my instincts were correct: I had PCOS.

My blood work came back with elevated insulin and lutenizing hormone, and androgen levels so high that Dr. Sherif, who is Middle Eastern, remarked that if she had my levels she would probably have a full beard. I, for some reason, am not prone to excessive hair growth. It also turned out I was deficient in vitamin D. I started taking metformin for the elevated insulin and soon started experiencing fewer cravings for carbohydrates. I cut back slightly on my carbohydrate intake and made sure the grains I was eating were always whole. Although my weight did not change much, after a year of insulin-lowering medication and changes in my diet, I was able to get my insulin levels into normal ranges and my lipid panel had greatly improved. My husband and I conceived our first child with no difficulty one year after I was diagnosed with PCOS and started treatment.

Although my symptoms weren't typical, my instinct that I had PCOS was strong, driving my search for answers. This book is written to give you, the dietitian, the knowledge and training needed to recognize PCOS among your clients (or even yourselves). It is my hope that you use this knowledge to provide effective medical nutrition therapy to help women improve their symptoms, prevent further medical complications, and live better lives.

Angela Grassi, MS, RD, LDN

FOR CHRIS

CHAPTER 1

UNDERSTANDING PCOS

BY KATHERINE. D. SHERIF, MD, FACP

WHAT CAUSES PCOS?

POLYCYSTIC OVARY SYNDROME (PCOS) affects 10% of women in the U.S. and is the most common cause of menstrual irregularities and infertility. PCOS has been viewed as solely a collection of reproductive health problems, including polycystic ovaries, irregular periods, infertility, and miscarriage associated with hirsutism, acne and overweight. However, PCOS is also associated with risk factors for heart disease.

Many women with PCOS have female relatives on either the maternal or paternal side with a history of irregular periods and/ or infertility. PCOS appears to be polygenic; multiple types of gene mutations seem to cause similar symptoms. In the past, an abnormal hypothalamic-pituitary-ovarian axis was identified as the basic etiology. However, it has become clearer that insulin plays a central role in the pathophysiology. Women with PCOS are insulin resistant: the resulting hyperinsulinemia stimulates ovarian insulin receptors, which in turn causes the ovaries to produce greater-than-normal amounts of testosterone. The testosterone, in turn, inhibits ovulation and causes the androgenic symptoms.

Insulin resistance → hyperinsulinemia → ovarian insulin receptors →↑↑ testosterone

PCOS symptoms can be attributed to two underlying processes: hyperinsulinemia and hyperandrogenemia. Hyperinsulinemia, as a potent growth hormone, is associated with weight gain. Weight gain causes insulin resistance and subsequent hyperinsulinemia, which in turns causes weight gain. The vicious cycle of insulin resistance makes it possible to gain weight very easily despite good nutrition and exercise. Hyperinsulinemia causes acanthosis nigricans, which is Latin for "black skin." In people with dark skin, hyperinsulinemia is easy to detect as dark soft skin on the back of the neck, the elbows, knees, underarms, between the breasts, across the knuckles and groin. In people with lighter skin, acanthosis nigricans may manifest as tan-appearing skin above the neckline and rough grey elbows. Hyperinsulinemia also causes skin tags and follicular keratosis, reddened rough hair follicles on the upper arms. The greater the hyperinsulinemia, the more severe the acanthosis nigricans.

The other symptoms are caused by high androgens, primarily testosterone, produced by the ovaries. They include irregular menstrual cycles and infertility. Other androgenic symptoms include severe acne and hirsutism of the face, jaw, chest, lower abdomen, or upper shoulders. One of the most distressing symptoms that women report is androgenic alopecia, or diffuse loss of scalp hair.

Women with PCOS also have a higher incidence of miscarriages, preterm deliveries, and stillbirths, but it is not clear whether these problems stem from high testosterone or high insulin.

CONDITIONS ASSOCIATED WITH PCOS

In addition to the symptoms described above, PCOS is associated with many other conditions which worsen health. These include an increased risk for endometrial cancer, which may result from irregular, uncontrolled bleeding. Other associations include obstructive sleep apnea which not only results from obesity, but from high testosterone which may cause apnea through a central brain mechanism. Depression is common in PCOS, which may compound overweight by causing a lack of motivation to eat well and exercise. Women with PCOS are also four times more likely to develop hypothyroidism, which is associated with fatigue, depression, weight gain and alopecia.

Recently, PCOS has been identified with multiple cardiovascular risk factors, including:

- Hypertension
- Hyperlipidemia
    - Hypertriglyceridemia
    - Low HDL
- Abnormal carbohydrate metabolism, including
    - insulin resistance
    - impaired fasting glucose
    - type 2 diabetes
- Metabolic syndrome
- Coagulopathy
- Hypothyroidism, recently recognized as a risk factor, is associated with high LDL

In retrospective international studies, women with irregular menstrual cycles are more likely to develop coronary artery disease at younger ages than women with regular cycles, even if the woman was not identified as having PCOS.

DIAGNOSIS

The absence of definitive criteria for PCOS have made it difficult to diagnose and especially difficult to compare studies. The most recent agreed-upon definition was developed by the European Society for Human Reproduction & the American Society for Reproductive Medicine in 2003. They define PCOS as two out of the three following:

1. irregular periods
2. hyperandrogenemic symptoms or elevated serum androgens
3. polycystic ovaries by transvaginal ultrasound

HISTORY

The patient's history is the most important element in the diagnosis of PCOS, followed by physical examination and blood tests. The typical history reveals menarche at the average of 12 to 13 years. Almost immediately, menses occur at irregular intervals. Often, teenagers will be told that irregular menses are a normal part of development and that they will grow out of it. At this point, girls are often prescribed oral contraceptive pills to initiate regular menses prior to the establishment of a diagnosis. Oral contraceptives result in lower serum androgen levels, decreased ovarian androgen production, and improvements in menstrual cyclicity, hirsutism, and acne, and in fact form a mainstay of therapy. However, hormonal contraceptives may delay diagnosis because the teen may now report regular menses. After a period of some years, these women often discontinue the oral contraceptive, perhaps to conceive and resume a pattern of irregular menses. It is at this point that they often turn to a gynecologist, perhaps blaming the oral contraceptives for their menstrual irregularity and infertility rather than addressing the underlying condition that led to the requirement hormonal contraception in the first place.

PHYSICAL EXAMINATION

After the history, the next most important component in the diagnosis of PCOS is the physical examination. Vital signs may be notable for an elevated blood pressure in the 130's/80's. Most women and girls with PCOS have central obesity consisting of fat deposition in the abdomen, upper arms and upper back. The diagnosis of PCOS may be overlooked in girls who are slender.

Hirsutism may or may not be present on the chin, neck, cheeks, chest, periareolar area, upper arms, back, or abdomen. Even if there are only a few terminal hairs on the chest, between the breasts, or on the lower abdomen, hair in these areas are indicative of elevated serum androgens. Acne may be non-existent, mild or severe, and may be present on the face, neck, upper arms, upper chest, back or buttocks. Diffuse alopecia is common.

Extensive abdominal striations, a buffalo hump, facial plethora and very thin limbs in contrast to abdominal obesity should prompt a work up for Cushing's disease.

It is important to remember that not all women with PCOS have all the above symptoms! The phenotypic presentations are variable because the etiology is probably multifactorial. For example, some women may not have the testosterone receptors in skin that cause hirsutism, especially women of East Asian descent. Other women may have a normal body mass index (BMI) of less than 25 and still have PCOS. Some women do not have acne or alopecia. A very small minority will have regular menses, but have most of the other features of hyperandrogenism and polycystic ovaries. The absence of all classically-described symptoms should not automatically exclude PCOS.

LABORATORY VALUES

It is important to note that blood values obtained while a patient is on the oral contraceptive pill (OCP) are not useful in diagnosing PCOS. Patients should be off the OCP for at least six weeks before measuring hormone levels. The most useful lab test in the work-up of PCOS is a total testosterone. A total testosterone > 50ng/dL is considered elevated. Free testosterone is a less reliable measurement. Other confirmatory labs include a luteinizing hormone (LH) to follicle stimulating hormone (FSH) ratio of greater than 2 or 3. Serum insulin measurements can be helpful to rule in insulin resistance. A normal insulin level is considered to be below 10. However, a blood specimen used to analyze serum insulin must be frozen quickly and in a typical office setting, it may not be frozen quickly enough, or may be allowed to thaw on the way to the lab. This results in erroneously low insulin levels. An oral glucose tolerance test may be ordered, although in most women with PCOS, it is obvious that they are insulin resistant due to central obesity and acanthosis nigricans.

There are few other conditions which cause irregular menstrual cycles, but they must be ruled out before making the diagnosis of PCOS. All women with a history of irregular menses should have the following initial tests: pregnancy test, prolactin level (to rule out a prolactin-secreting pituitary adenoma) and thyroid-stimulating hormone (TSH) (to rule out hypo- or hyperthyroidism). Other tests can be performed depending on the clinical presentation:

- Cushing's disease in a patient with moon fascies, buffalo hump, central obesity and abdominal striae and very thin arms and legs in relation to obesity.
  o Check a 24-hour urine for cortisol
- Androgen-secreting tumour in a patient with sudden virilizing symptoms
  o Check DHEA-sulfate (not DHEA)
- Late-onset (or "non-classical") congenital adrenal hyperplasia in a woman of Greek, Jewish, Latina or Italian descent with precocious puberty
  o Check a DNA test for common mutations of the 21-hydroxylase gene

A fasting lipid profile is useful for assessing cardiovascular risk. The typical pattern in insulin resistant or diabetic patients is elevated triglycerides and decreased HDL. After treatment is begun, it is helpful to repeat blood tests in three to six months to assess the change in testosterone and improvement in lipid profile. A list of lab tests used to diagnose and monitor PCOS can be found in Table. 1.

Table 1. List of lab tests to diagnose and monitor PCOS
Fasting Insulin
Total testosterone
Free testosterone
Luteinizing hormone (LH)
Follicle stimulating hormone (FSH)
DHEA-sulfate (not DHEA)
Prolactin
17 alpha-hydroxyprogesterone
Thyroid stimulating hormone (TSH)
Liver function tests
Fasting lipid profile
Fasting chemistry (which includes glucose)

TRANSVAGINAL SONOGRAPHY

Transvaginal sonography (TVS) is necessary for infertility evaluation and management. However, if a patient does not wish to conceive, and if she has a classic history and signs of PCOS, a TVS without evidence of polycystic ovaries probably would not change management. The classic PCOS finding on TVS is a "string of pearls", which describes typical cysts that are peripheral, multiple and less than 10mm in diameter.

MEDICAL TREATMENT OF PCOS

Medications include hormonal contraception, androgen blockers and insulin sensitizers. Office visits should be about every three months to evaluate the effect of medications, especially in the beginning. The most commonly used medication for PCOS is the oral contraceptive pill (OCP). The supraphysiologic doses of estrogen suppress FSH and LH and induce regular periods. Estrogen also increases sex hormone binding globulin in the liver which binds free testosterone, making it unavailable to tissues. Acne may improve dramatically, and hirsutism and alopecia often decrease. However, OCPs may not cause sufficient improvement in metabolic parameters and may increase insulin resistance.

Spironolactone is a weak antihypertensive medication that is effective for hirsutism and alopecia. Spironolactone, an androgen blocker, competes with testosterone for androgen receptors. Spironolactone may be used alone or in combination with other medications. Although it may take months to see an effect, the improvement in alopecia can be striking. Spironolactone is so weak as a blood pressure-lowering medication that patients rarely, if ever, experience hypotension. *The main caution with this drug is that it is a potent teratogen and must not be used in women who may become pregnant.*

Metformin, an insulin sensitizer, can help patients surmount hyperinsulinemia, especially in conjunction with healthy diet and exercise. Through its effect on lowering insulin levels, metformin aids weight loss, decreases testosterone levels, induces ovulation, improves lipid profile and lowers blood pressure. Metformin is safe in pregnancy and has been shown to decrease first-trimester miscarriages that are common in PCOS. Since metformin is commonly associated with gastrointestinal effects such as nausea, bloating and diarrhea, it should be titrated up slowly and taken after meals. Patients need to be reminded that metformin is so effective in inducing ovulation that if they do not want to conceive, they must use contraception, even if they never have before.

Ovarian drilling is an old method of surgically reducing the size of the ovaries, which are enlarged in PCOS. By decreasing the mass of the ovaries, less androgens are produced. Although ovarian drilling can be effective in improving symptoms in PCOS, it is no longer considered the treatment of choice.

FUTURE FRONTIERS

Although obesity confers insulin resistance, insulin resistance is more severe in obese women with PCOS compared to obese women without PCOS. The vicious cycle of obesity, insulin resistance and further obesity is accelerated in PCOS. Treatment of PCOS should be focus on improving understanding of the genetic basis of insulin resistance. Insulin resistance worsens with age, so the other priority should be earlier diagnosis and treatment of adolescents.

In summary, PCOS, a leading cause of menstrual irregularities and infertility, is also associated with obesity, hirsutism and cardiovascular risk factors such as elevated blood pressure, hyperlipidemia and impaired glucose tolerance. Diagnosis is based on history of menstrual dysfunction and evidence of hyperandrogenemia. Insulin resistance appears to play a central role in the pathophysiology. Treatment is comprised of physical activity, proper nutrition and weight loss. OCPs induce monthly menstrual cycles and improve acne and hirsutism. Insulin sensitizers, such as metformin, induce ovulation and improve metabolic parameters. Insulin sensitizers play an important role in PCOS-associated infertility. Research should focus on understanding the etiology of the severe insulin resistance seen in PCOS.

REFERENCES

Balen A, Michelmore K. What is Polycystic Ovary Syndrome? *Hum Repro* 17(9): 2219-2227, 2002.

Deaton MA, Glorioso JE, McLean DB. Congenital adrenal hyperplasia: not really a zebra. *Amer Fam Physician* 59(5):1190-6, 1999.

Dunaif A. Insulin resistance and the polycystic ovary syndrome: mechanism and implications for pathogenesis. Endocr Rev 18:774-800, 1997.

Dunaif A, Segal KR, Futterweit W, Dobrjansky A. Profound peripheral insulin resistance, independent of obesity, in polycystic ovary syndrome. *Diabetes* 38:1165-1174, 1989.

Garber AJ. Duncan TJ, Goodman AM, Mills DJ, Rohlf JL. Efficacy of metformin in type 2 diabetes: results of a double-blind, placebo-controlled, dose-response trial. *Amer J Med* 103(6):491-7, 1997.

Lord JM, Flight IHK, Norman RJ. Metformin in polycystic ovary syndrome: systematic review and meta-analysis. *BMJ* 327:951, 2003.

Luthold WW. Borges MF. Marcondes JA. Hakohyama M. Wajchenberg BL. Kirschner MA. Serum testosterone fractions in women: normal and abnormal clinical states. *Metab Clin Exper* 42(5):638-43,1993.

Nelson VL, Legro RS, Strauss JF, McAllister JM. Augmented androgen production is a stable steroidogenic phenotype of propagated theca cells from polycystic ovaries. *Mol Endocrinol* 13:946-957, 1999.

Rebar R, Judd HL, Yen SS, Rakoff J, Vandenberg G, Naftolin F. Characterization of the inappropriate gonadotropin secretion in polycystic ovarian syndrome. *J Clin Invest* 57:1320-1329, 1976.

Sherif K, Kushner H, Falkner BE. Sex hormone-binding globulin and insulin resistance in African-American women. *Metab Clin Experim* 47(1):70-4, 1998.

Sherif K. Benefits and risks of oral contraceptives. *Amer J Obstet Gyn* 180(6):S343-8, 1999.

Zawedzki JK, Dunaif A. Diagnostic criteria for polycystic ovary syndrome: towards a rational approach. In: Dunaif A, Givens JR, Haseltine FP, Merriam GR, Eds. *Polycystic ovary syndrome:* Boston: Glasckwell Scientific; 377-384, 1992.

CHAPTER 2

THE PSYCHOLOGICAL ASPECTS OF PCOS

BY STEPHANIE B. MATTEI, PSY.D.
AND
MICHELLE SHWARZ, MSED

JULIE IS THIRTEEN. SHE began menstruating two years ago, but without any regularity. Recently, she has noticed some unusual things happening to her body that do not seem to be happening to her friends. She is concerned about the extra hair sprouting on her chest, on her belly, and on her face. She is covered in acne and is a bit concerned that she is somewhat heavier than her peers. Julie, embarrassed, asks her mother to take her to the doctor. Her mother tells her that she will grow out of it and believes that Julie is experiencing normal adolescent worries about her new developing body. In the meantime, she starts waxing the unwanted hair and secretly starts to skip breakfast and lunch in hopes that her belly will go away. She struggles to concentrate and focus on her schoolwork. All she can think about is how abnormal she looks and feels. These thoughts are consuming her at school and in public. The only solace she has is alone in her room.

At fifteen, she is still not getting her period on any regular basis; twice a year at best with much monthly spotting. This irregularity is causing her some additional anxiety since she never knows when she will get her period, or when the spotting will just "show up." Additionally, Julie is heavier still. Her fasting diet has slipped into a fasting/binging cycle, which is contributing to feelings of guilt, shame and the thoughts that she is inferior to her thinner peers. She finally convinces her mother to take her to the doctor, who subsequently tells Julie to stop eating junk food and to watch what she is consuming because she is borderline obese. The doctor prescribes birth control pills. Resentful of the doctor's diet advice but relieved to get some hope of normalcy, Julie starts the pill and finally gets her monthly period with extreme predictability and her acne virtually clears up.

Her mother takes her to the endocrinologist who lets her know that her slightly elevated testosterone is just part of puberty. However, Julie and her mother often have conversations about her coming off the pill, because her mother secretly fears that Julie now has permission to have sex. There is strain in their relationship and Julie feels even more isolated. Her mother and family, which were once the source of support, are now the source of even more stress. Julie is cranky and irritable most of the time, but again her mother brushes it off as a normal teenaged stage.

In addition, the pounds come piling on, sometimes 10 lbs per month. In one year Julie had gone from 180 pounds and size 14 to 260 pounds and size 22. She is devastated that she no longer can shop at the trendy stores that her girlfriends are getting their cute clothes. She starts losing her confidence that she would ever have the opportunity to date in high school, let alone be in an intimate relationship or have sex. Her low-self esteem becomes the resounding factor by which Julie is defining herself. Julie is depressed; she no longer just has teenage blues. She withdraws from her peer group, no longer participates in her favorite activities, and eating and sleeping become her primary activities out of school.

Julie is now thirty-two and has met the love of her life seven years ago. During the past seventeen years, Julie has cycled in and out of her depression. Her weight has fluctuated by 50 or more pounds per year, but gratefully, she is acne free and gets her period every month on "the Pill." She is quite heavy-set but her sweetheart believes her to be quite beautiful. Despite his clear attraction to her, she is not quite as sexually comfortable and satisfied as she would like. Julie and her husband decide to start a family, and for the first time in more than a decade and a half, she comes off the pill. After the first few months,

Julie does not get her period and excitedly takes a pregnancy test, but receives a negative result. After two weeks, she still does not get her period and retakes the home test, again with negative results. After trying to become pregnant for six months, Julie finally confides in her husband that she has not had her period for that entire time. Her mood shifts from depressed to irritable; she is angry and frustrated for more days than not. Frustrated, the couple goes to see a fertility specialist for a consultation. After taking a full history, the doctor performs an intra-vaginal ultrasound confirming the presence of ovarian cysts. He confirms the diagnosis of PCOS.

While the physical symptoms of (PCOS) are becoming increasingly recognized in the medical world, the psychological effects are lagging in recognition. The following chapter is a review of the various issues that women with PCOS might experience. Issues about body image and self-esteem arise out of abnormal stress responses that correlate with significant weight gain: hirsutism (excess hair growth on the face and body), acne, infertility problems and issues with sex-drive. Eating disorders, depression, anxiety and bipolar disorder are also common clinical conditions observed in these women. Lastly, recommendations for treatment and appropriate professional referrals will aid the dietitian in noticing when an issue as arisen, as well as how to steer these patients in the direction to get the help they need.

BODY IMAGE AND SELF ESTEEM

Much like Julie, women with PCOS may feel shameful about their bodies and the various medical conditions they experience. They may feel ashamed that they cannot control their weight through exercise or diet, or because they have hair growing on their face and body that they do not like. Sexually active women could be concerned that they may be pregnant because there are no obvious guides to let them know when they are ovulating. Furthermore, many physicians and other health care professionals are still undereducated about the complexities of PCOS, and as a result, they may give "supportive" advice to their PCOS patients such as to lose weight or "don't worry," which only contribute to the urges to isolate and engage in poor coping choices.

Most women in American society correlate their body image with self-esteem. Ironically, a person's actual size or appearance may not directly correlate with their body image. Someone who is perceived unattractive by others may have a positive body image, whereas someone who is perceived as attractive by others may have negative self-image. Self-image is a valuation that someone places on themselves and what they have to offer. It encompasses more than just body image; it might also include perceived intelligence, kindness, altruism, and personality all play a part in shaping self-image.

Women with PCOS may overlook these aspects and consider body image more important in forming self-image. They might desire a particular body shape or size and have emotions about their ability to either achieve it. Himelein and Thatcher (1) note the increased negative body image in women diagnosed with PCOS compared to counterparts who have similar body compositions. In fact, women with PCOS exceed both "control group women and national test norms on measures of body dissatisfaction" (2).

STRESS RESPONSES AND WEIGHT

Stress is a given in the complicated lives of women today, and there has been a plethora of research into the impact stress has on human beings. With "stress management" being an everyday phrase in today's society, the stress response in humans vary in as many ways as there are possibilities of stressful events. Americans engage in numerous unhealthy behaviors as a way of self-soothing from their stresses. According to a national survey conducted by the American Psychological Association, some of these behaviors to deal with stress are comfort eating, poor diet choices, smoking and inactivity (3). People experiencing stress are more likely to report hypertension, anxiety or depression and obesity. According to this survey (3), "women report feeling the effects of stress on their physical health more than men. The survey results seem to tie in with what research shows, that 43 percent of all adults suffer adverse health effects from stress. Given the potential health complications related to stress, it is fair to say stress certainly is a health problem in America."

For women with PCOS, there is more. Not only is there the

"typical" stress reaction, but there may be additional responses due the hormonal impact of the condition. A study done by Rutledge and Linden (4) showed that women who are restrictive eaters tend to increase their food consumption under stress as opposed to non-restrictive eaters. This is an important finding for dietitians working with women with PCOS who are focusing on monitoring and regulating the food consumption. Women with PCOS may engage in more excessive eating than those women without the diagnosis.

In addition, because of the potential amplified physiological affect of stress on PCOS women, the stress-eat reaction may last longer than for women without the diagnosis. Epel et al (5) studied fifty-nine healthy pre-menopausal women to determine the effect that stress has on eating behavior. The women were observed in both stress and control conditions. The research found that those women in the stress condition who had higher cortisol levels also had a higher caloric intake, as opposed to those with lower cortisol levels who had lower caloric intake. Interestingly enough, during the non-stress condition, both groups ate similar amounts. Additionally, the higher cortisol group ate more "sweet foods" than did the lower cortisol group. Another interesting finding of the study showed that "increases in negative mood in response to the stressors were also significantly related to greater food consumption" (5). These findings suggest that stress and increased eating behavior may be part of a vicious perpetual cycle that may be difficult for women with PCOS to combat, due to the fact that these women produce more of the stress hormone cortisol under repeated stress.

HIRSUTISM AND DERMATOLOGICAL ISSUES

Symptoms like hirsutism, or excessive hair growth in women in locations where the occurrence of hair is normally minimal or absent, contribute to the increase in stress for women diagnosed with PCOS. They are likely to see themselves as "unfeminine" or even monstrous. More than 70% of women with PCOS complain of symptoms such as hair loss, or hair growth, on the face, back, stomach, chest, thumbs or toes. Lipton et al (6) studied eighty-eight women with facial hair and found that two thirds of them (67%) continually checked themselves in the mirror, with 76% of them checking with touch. On average, these women spent 104 minutes a week, managing this hair. Hirsutism, in addition to acne and oily skin, are caused by the high androgen levels that women with PCOS have.

Acne and oily skin, especially at an early age, can influence self-esteem greatly. Being overly concerned with appearance at any age can be problematic, but teens and young women especially have the added worry of being concerned with how others see them. This pre-occupation with being "normal" or "pretty" to others not only influences and contributes to negative body image, but also influences the manner in which these girls and women interact with their environment, with people and the world. These women might be shy in social environments, isolative, and even might develop anxiety related to social events.

IRREGULAR MENSES, SEX DRIVE AND INFERTILITY

Irregular menses, unusual sex drive and issues with fertility can also contribute to low self-esteem (7). With minimal education around the diagnosis and detection of PCOS, young women with difficult and irregular menstrual cycles are left feeling confused and often scared. Much like we saw with Julie, they do not understand what is happening to their bodies, why their periods are so heavy, abnormal, or non-existent, or even more importantly, why this is happening to them. Consequently, life-long feelings of shame, frustration, failure, and guilt can lead anyone to have reduced self-esteem that impacts body image.

Women with PCOS also experience issues with sex drive that women without this diagnosis do not typically experience. Trent, Rich and Austin (8) studied sexual behavior in adolescent girls with PCOS and discovered that these girls engage in sexual relationships later than their non-PCOS counterparts. Himelein & Thatcher (1) hypothesize that this may be due to their perceived lower sexual desirability. When this trend was investigated, a strong correlation between perceived sexual attraction, body image and sexual satisfaction was found. Women with PCOS believed that their sexual partners weren't as satisfied with them as did women without PCOS (9). Hirsutism, acne, and other superficial factors were also linked to sexual satisfaction and social outgoingness.

It has been hypothesized that women diagnosed with PCOS have a higher sexual desire than other women because of the increase in male hormones. Several studies have dispelled this belief, and in fact have showed that women with PCOS had a decrease in sexual desire and perceived sexual attractiveness, and that libido did not correlate at all with androgen levels (9,10,).

Infertility, the most common medical complication associated with PCOS, occurs in approximately 75% of women who have been diagnosed with PCOS due to anovulation (11). The feelings of loss, grief, depression and even anxiety that come with the desire to become pregnant and the inability to do so can be devastating. Women who are experiencing this often ruminate or think about their infertility issues more often than not, and in fact, they have difficulty concentrating or thinking about anything else. Additionally, symptoms of depression such as anhedonia, or diminished pleasure in activities that were once enjoyable, social isolation, or even thoughts about death or suicide might present themselves. The impact of this dilemma, left unattended, can lead to debilitating dysfunction in the women diagnosed with PCOS and the destruction of even the best relationships.

CLINICAL CONDITIONS

Other psychological effects that women diagnosed with PCOS may struggle with are the clinical conditions that would need to be treated with the assistance of a mental health professional. These syndromes: Binge Eating Disorder, Bulimia, Major Depressive Disorder, Bipolar Disorder, and Anxiety will be described briefly as well as how they may affect the woman diagnosed with PCOS. If, as a dietitian, you suspect that one of your patients may be suffering from one of the aforementioned conditions, it is imperative that you ascertain the opinion of a psychiatrist, psychologist, or other mental health professional to acquire an appropriate diagnosis. These conditions, which can be treated successfully with empirically supported treatments, should be approached by the entire clinical treatment team as significant as the PCOS diagnosis (12,13).

Figure 1: Binge Eating Disorder and
Bulimia Nervosa Diagnostic Flow Chart (16)

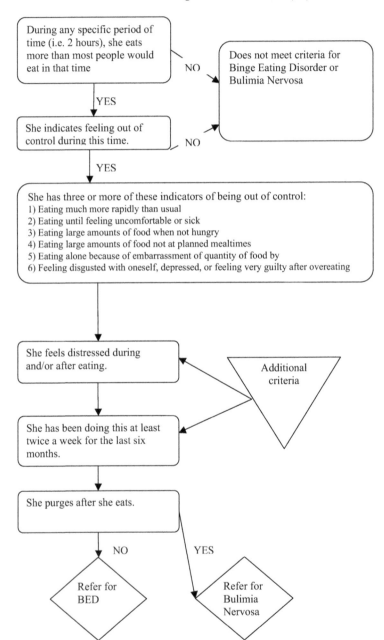

BINGE EATING DISORDER AND BULIMIA NERVOSA

Stress eating, overeating, and binge eating disorder are often confused. Binge eating disorder (BED) is currently being evaluated by the American Psychiatric Association to determine if it should be included into the next Diagnostic and Statistical Manual (14). According the APA, Binge eating disorder would include "recurrent episodes of binge eating associated with subjective and behavioral indicators of impaired control, and significant distress about, the binge eating and the absence of the regular use of inappropriate compensatory behaviors (such as self induced vomiting, misuse of laxatives and other medications, fasting, and excessive exercises) that are characteristics of Bulimia Nervosa" (14).

As for prevalence, it states in the DSM-IV-TR (14) that "in samples drawn from weight control programs, the overall prevalence varies from approximately 15%-50%, with females approximately 1.5 times more likely to have this eating problem than males. In non-patient community samples, a prevalence rate of 0.7% - 4% has been reported." Other sources indicate that Binge eating disorder occurs in 2% of the population (15). Of importance is that while the non-patient prevalence is small, the percentage of patients seen by a dietitian is much higher, as it falls within the range of those patients seeking assistance for weight issues.

Figure 1 shows the process that an appropriate mental health professional might use in differentiating between BED and Bulimia Nervosa (15). The major difference between the two diagnoses is the compensatory behavior that occurs after a binge has occurred. While the dietitian may not be making the diagnosis, it is critical to understand the reasons for the difference in diagnosis.

Bulimia Nervosa (BN) is another eating disorder that is often found in women diagnosed with PCOS. BN is categorized by binge eating and inappropriate compensatory methods to prevent weight gain (14). There is a frequent co-morbidity with Mood Disorders in these patients. Often the mood disorder develops after the initial diagnosis of BN. While the details of BN in relationship to PCOS will be discussed further in this book, it is important for the dietitian to be mindful that there are empirically supported treatments for BN such as Cognitive Behavioral Therapy, and Interpersonal Therapy (12,13) that can assist these patients in the recovery process.

MAJOR DEPRESSION

Depression is a distinct psychological disorder that is different than the "blues" or "feeling down" that all people experience occasionally during their day-to-day lives. It is also different from a grief response that may result from the death of a loved one or the loss of a relationship. Depression is an overwhelming experience that depletes an individual or energy, interest in activities that once gave them pleasure, and can be recurring throughout an individual's life.

Major Depression Disorder (MDD) is diagnosed when an individual has experienced one or more Major Depressive Episodes, without a history of Manic, Mixed, or Hypomanic episodes. The individual must have experienced a significant change in functioning, where one of the major clinical manifestations is either (1) depressed mood, or (2) loss of interest of pleasure (3). In order for a Major Depressive Episode to be diagnosed, at least five of the following symptoms need to be present during a two-week period:

(1) Depressed mood most of the day, nearly every day, as indicated by either subjective report (e.g. feels sad or empty) or observation made by others (e.g. appears tearful) **Note:** In children and adolescents, can be irritable mood.

(2) Markedly diminished interest or pleasure in all, or almost all, activities most of the day, nearly every day (as indicated by either subjective account or observation made by others).

(3) Significant weight loss when not dieting, or weight gain (e.g. a change of more than 5% of body weight in a month), or decrease or increase in appetite nearly every day. **Note:** In children, consider failure to make expected weight gains.

(4) Insomnia or hypersomnia nearly day.

(5) Psychomotor agitation or retardation nearly every day (observable by others, not merely subjective feelings of restlessness or being slowed down)

(6) Fatigue or loss of energy every day.

(7) Feelings of worthlessness or excessive or inappropriate guilt

(which may be delusional) nearly every day (not merely self-reproach or guilt about being sick).

(8) Diminished ability to think or concentrate, or indecisiveness, nearly every day (either by subjective account or as observed by others).

(9) Recurrent thoughts of death (not just fear of dying), recurrent suicidal ideation without a specific plan, or a suicide attempt of a specific plan for committing suicide.

Other criteria for the diagnosis attend to differentiating depression from other diagnoses, as well as noting areas in the individual's life that have been impaired. It is important for the dietitian to note that patients who experience depression will often report feelings of sadness, feeling down, tearfulness, and general unhappiness (14).

The relationship between MDD and PCOS is well documented (1,2,16,17). Due to the increase in androgen production, women with PCOS are at greater risk for a depressive episode. To understand the connection between PCOS and androgen production, it is essential to grasp the connection between androgens and insulin. "Hyperandrogenism in PCOS can be the result of androgen overproduction by the adrenals as well as the ovaries, and in turn, it can lead to hyperinsulinemia and insulin resistance" (16). An increase in insulin resistance has been associated with depression. Insulin also affects serotonin (a neurotransmitter that plays an important role in depression, aggression, anger, sexuality, body temperature and appetite) levels. Dysregulated serotonin is a leading cause in depression (16).

It is interesting to note that many women with PCOS who are prescribed oral contraceptive medication have a different response in relationship to depression, as do women without PCOS diagnosis. That is, women with PCOS often experience a decrease in depression while taking oral contraceptives. This relationship is interesting because the use of oral contraception has been related to insulin resistance in other studies (18).

Brown (19) reviewed the literature concerning the co-morbid occurrence of insulin resistant disorders, such as diabetes and depression, to strengthen the hypothesis of the insulin-resistant cause for depression in PCOS patients. She points to a study that shows improvements in insulin sensitivity when non-insulin resistant depressed patients were treated with antidepressants (20). This study (21) encourages longer and larger scale studies of co-morbid depression and insulin sensitivity disorders to better understand this relationship. Furthermore, it has been hypothesized but insufficiently tested, that insulin-sensitizing medications, such as metformin (glucophage®, Bristol-Myers Squibb Co.), can improve depression symptoms.

While the insulin resistance hypothesis for depression in women diagnosed with PCOS is strong, it excludes the lean women diagnosed with PCOS and those with PCOS who do not have insulin resistance. Keegan et al (22) examined depression symptoms in non-overweight and non-obese PCOS patients with hirsutism. They found a strong presence of depression in these women, which was higher than their comparison group of patients with cancer. Weight-matched controlled studies (1,2) have shown a continued increased prevalence of depression in PCOS women compared to normal controls, regardless of whether the women with PCOS was lean or obese.

There are hypotheses about the origins of depression in women diagnosed with PCOS other than those related to insulin resistance. Weiner et al (23) compared mood states between PCOS patients and normally menstruating women. They found a relationship between free testosterone (FT) and depression, with women who were diagnosed with PCOS experiencing more acute and long standing depressive symptoms than women with normal hormone levels. In addition, other mood state differences including hostility and anxiety were linked to increased free testosterone in women diagnosed with PCOS (23).

BIPOLAR DISORDERS

Bipolar I disorder, once called Manic Depression, is diagnosed when a client has a history of both depressive and manic episodes. A person who is pleasure seeking, fast paced and an increased rate of speech stereotypically portrays the disorder. A Bipolar I diagnosis is given when the individual has experienced at least one or more Manic Episodes or Mixed Episodes. While individuals might also have experienced a Major Depressive Episode, its presence is not necessary for the diagnosis.

A Manic Episode is characterized by a distinct period of time (at least one week) in which there is an abnormally and persistently elevated, expansive or irritated mood (14). At least three or more of the following symptoms must also accompany the mood disturbance:

(1)   Inflated self-esteem or grandiosity
(2)   Decreased need for sleep (e.g. feels rested after only 3 hours of sleep)
(3)   More talkative than usual or pressure to keep talking
(4)   Flight of ideas of subjective experience that thoughts are racing
(5)   Distractibility (i.e. attention too easily drawn to unimportant or irrelevant external stimuli)
(6)   Increase in goal-directed activity (either socially, at work or school, or sexually) or psychomotor agitation
(7)   Excessive involvement in pleasurable activities that have a high potential for painful consequences (e.g. engaging in unrestrained buying sprees, sexual indiscretions, or foolish business investments).

There is another form of the disorder called Bipolar II disorder. Bipolar II disorder differs from Bipolar I disorder in that rather than having a manic episode, the patient has a history of at least one Hypomanic episode. The symptoms of hypomania are the same as mania; however, symptoms last from 4-6 days rather than lasting for one week. Irritability is also more likely to be the key mood during hypomania rather than elevated mood, and the disturbance is not severe enough to cause marked impairment. That is, during a hypomanic episode, there would be no need for hospitalization (14).

If you suspect that your client may have a Bipolar Disorder, it is important to refer them to a mental health specialist for an appropriate assessment and diagnosis. Bipolar disorder is often diagnosed over a period of time after evaluating a personal and family history as well as watching her symptoms over time.

In your office, you might notice someone in a manic or hypomanic episode. You may observe that the rate or speed of their speech has increased, that she interrupts you often, or it may seem like you have difficulty getting her to stop talking. When she does talk, they may talk in non-sequiturs. That is, she may bounce from topic to topic without a logic progression of thoughts and it might seem quite tangential. Keeping her attention could also be more difficult or you may find her focusing on details that are irrelevant. She may tell you about specific new plans that they may have involving new business ventures, having children, starting or ending relationships, etc. Finally, her pleasure seeking behavior is significantly different than what people without bipolar disorder would participate in. Rather, the behaviors that she engages in may have serious consequences, such as going on a spending spree, engaging in promiscuous sex, or suddenly quitting her job.

While these symptoms describe more of the clichéd manic episode, mania may present differently in the PCOS woman. Particularly, whereas elevated mood, grandiosity, and hyperactivity may be the most notable symptoms of the aforementioned form of mania, women diagnosed with PCOS may present with irritability instead of elevated mood as the main feature of their mania.

As a dietitian working with women diagnosed with PCOS, it is very likely that you will come across a patient with either an undiagnosed or diagnosed bipolar disorder. This is because of the high correlation between the two diagnoses. While there are numerous explanations as to why this is so, one theory states that the "antiepileptic drugs (AED) used to treat bipolar disorder, especially valproate, may indirectly promote PCOS" (1,17). Valproate, or Depakote is a commonly prescribed mood stabilizer. As for mechanism of action, Himelein and Thatcher (1) note that research is pointing to the effect that prolonged exposure to valproate has on the ovaries. That is, that there is an increased ovarian androgen biosynthesis when there has been sustained exposure to valproate.

Joffe and collegues (24) corroborated these findings; 34.2% of women with bipolar disorder, 24.5% of women with depression, and 21.7% of healthy female controls had reported early onset of menstrual cycle dysfunction. Women with bipolar disorder, therefore, are 1.7 times more likely to have menstrual disturbances versus healthy controls. Additionally, while larger studies have no shown higher rates of PCOS in the general population, menstrual abnormalities have been noted.

Another theory suggests that there is a connection between bipolar disorders and PCOS that is independent of valproate or other anti-epileptic drugs (25). In fact, Kliptstein & Goldberg (25) state that there have been studies attempting to connect the use of valproate with an increase prevalence of PCOS. They have not found such an association. They found that while bipolar disorders are more prevalent in women with PCOS than in the general public, there was no connection to the use of valproate. These authors suggest "PCOS may inherently arise in a substantial minority of women with possible bipolar disorder, potentially via a shared hypothalamic-pi-tuitary- gonadal axis defect. Because bipolar illness has previously been linked with thyroid and adrenocortical endocrinopathesis, it is conceivable that hypothalamic-pituitary axis dysfunction could demarcate a biologically distinct bipolar subtype."

ANXIETY

Anxiety, or persistent worry, is a normal response to situations that are dangerous or scary. We are biologically "hard-wired" to experi-ence panic, anxiety, or fear when we are at risk for danger. Panic and anxiety protects us by initiating the autonomic nervous system or the "fight or flight" response. Some of the symptoms of fear that you might notice are:

(1)   Physiological, such as increased heart rate, sweating or dizziness
(2)   Cognitive, such as automatic thoughts about being abnormal or less than perfect
(3)   Motivational, such as the wish to be as far away from the dangerous situation as possible
(4)   Emotional, such as the feeling of fear or terror
(5)   Behavioral, such as nail biting or inhibited speech

In today's society, fear and anxiety are often used interchangeably (26). Fear typically refers to the appraisal that something unwanted or catastrophic is about to occur and the person is assessing the poten-tial danger ahead. As such, you can see how the aforementioned symptoms of fear would make sense. Anxiety, however, is something different. Anxiety is defined as a "tense emotional state that is often marked by such physical symptoms as tension, tremor, sweating and increased pulse rate (26). The two differ in that anxiety is an emotional experience and fear is a cognitive one. "Fear involves the intellectual appraisal of a stimuli, and anxiety involves the emotional response to the appraisal."

This distinction between fear and anxiety is critical. It is possible that the women diagnosed with PCOS might be afraid of particular social situations or other stimuli that she perceives as being potentially dangerous. Perhaps she is feeling vulnerable to danger, criticism, or being exposed. This fear, which might be justified for the person's situation and experience, may be difficult for others to understand and might be motivation for the individual to make certain life choices.

Anxiety on the other hand, is not necessarily based on an appraisal of a situation, but is an emotional experience that is based on something quite different. Often, anxiety is hallmarked by excessive and uncontrollable worry, which is based upon particular stimuli that the individual has attended to while choosing to ignore stimuli that may indicate that no danger is present (26).

Part of a normal stress response, fear and anxiety become problematic when they begin to impair an individual's ability to function. If your patient is experiencing worry about social situations but is not experiencing any impairment in her life, that is quite different than the patient who avoids leaving the house and cannot consequently live a life that is congruent with her goals. Anxiety comes in many forms such as Panic attacks, Agoraphobia, Posttraumatic Stress Disorder, Acute Stress Disorder, Social Anxiety, and Generalized Anxiety. If you are concerned that your patient might be experiencing a pathological or impairing amount of anxiety, please refer her to a mental health specialist for assessment.

TREATMENT FOR PSYCHOLOGICAL ISSUES

Psychological issues can be managed in many ways ranging from psychotherapy, psychopharmacology, and complementary and alternative medicine (CAM). Psychotherapy is a formal, interpersonal, unilateral, systematic, time limited relationship, which focuses its attention on individual's problematic behaviors, thoughts or feelings with efforts to create change in the individual. While there are numerous schools of thought or theories behind psychotherapy methods, strategies and techniques, there are many which have found empirical support in treating particular psychological disorders. In addition to "talk therapies," psychopharmacology has been successful in creating change in psychological conditions as well. Various medications have been found to be effective in treating anxiety disorders as well as mood disorders. Lastly, many women diagnosed with PCOS might seek out alternative treatments such as homeopathy or herbal supplements to assist them with their feelings and emotions. More information on these topics can be found in Chapter 5.

PSYCHOTHERAPY

As mentioned previously, Psychotherapy comes in a variety of forms. Within the past two decades, The American Psychological Association has undergone the enormous undertaking of ascertaining information related to psychotherapy efficacy (12). Through this process, a considerable amount of information was discovered about which psychotherapy treatments were effective for particular disorders, and which psychotherapy treatments showed promise. In addition, this movement in developing empirically supported treatments has motivated clinicians and researchers to conduct similar experiments in a continued effort to develop effective psychotherapies.

For the treatment of Depression, the Behavioral treatment of depression, Cognitive-Behavioral Treatment and Interpersonal Psychotherapy have found empirical support. For Anxiety and stress related disorders, Cognitive therapy for panic, Applied relaxation for panic, Exposure treatment for agoraphobia, Cognitive behavioral Therapy for Generalized Anxiety Disorder, Exposure for social phobia, Stress Inoculation Training for coping with stressors, Exposure and response prevention for Obsessive Compulsive Disorder, Exposure/ guided imagery for specific phobia, and Systematic desensitization for specific phobia have found empirical research. For Eating Disorders, Cognitive Behavioral treatment for Bulimia and Interpersonal Therapy for Bulimia has been found to be efficacious.

There are additional therapies that have been showing promise in the treatment literature. Marsha Linehan originally developed Dialectical Behavior Therapy (DBT), for the treatment of parasuicidal and suicidal women. Since its inception, it has undergone rigorous studies and has found an application for Bulimia and Binge Eating Disorder (27). DBT might be effective for women with PCOS as it would teach them how to be mindful of various internal and external stimuli in a nonjudgmental manner, while being able to engage in behavior that is effective for their life. Patients are taught how to identify behaviors that are interfering with their quality of life, as well as those that are life threatening. The woman with PCOS might find this aspect most helpful. She will learn how to "chain" situations and implement emotion regulation, interpersonal effectiveness, and distress tolerance strategies to create a life worth living.

Mindfulness-based stress reduction (MBSR) uses the concept of mindfulness meditation as a skill to reduce stress, both psychologically and physically. Developed by Jon Kabat-Zinn in 1979, this eight-week program has demonstrated remarkable change in job related stress, people with physical conditions such as heart disease and high blood pressure, as well as anxiety substance abuse. MBSR might be helpful for women with PCOS as it will teach them how to be mindful of their bodies, of their eating patterns, and about their state of being.

Lastly, support groups for women diagnosed with PCOS would be helpful as well. This type of group would ideally have a mental health professional as a group leader who would assist these patients in normalizing each others experiences and validating emotional responses that other significant people in their lives might not. In this group, these women can impart new information to each other about doctors and specialists as well as try out new interpersonal skills to aid them in the world. It would offer to them the opportunity to be part of a social network as well assist them in learning various new coping strategies. This concept of learning new coping strategies in dealing with the diagnosis, life changing behaviors and medications, as well as judgments that these patients might have is key.

PSYCHOPHARMACOLOGY

The field of psychopharmacology has expanded greatly over the past twenty years. With the advent of neuroscience and psychiatry, knowledge about psychiatric processes has grown exponentially. Medications for various psychological conditions are plentiful. For those prescribing medications, the process of observing symptoms, assessing the course of illness, and evaluating the risk-to benefit ratio is critical (28).

Medications for mood disorders come in different classes. Antidepressants such as elavil or wellbutrin are tricyclics and heterocyclics, while prozac and zoloft are SSRI's. Each of these medications has a different mechanism of action, and different adverse reactions. Another class of antidepressants is the MAOI inhibitors like parnate and nardil.

Mood stabilizers are primarily used for bipolar disorders. The most common of these are lithium carbonate and lamotrigine (lamictal). As mentioned earlier, some of these mood stabilizers have been thought to cause PCOS symptoms. In any case, most of these medications have potential side effects that may influence insulin resistance, weight gain, and weight loss. Of note is that is a current theory that insulin-sensitizing medications such as metformin may also help mood disorders in women with PCOS even though there is no current research evidence to supportive of this conjecture.

Medications for anxiety are also available. These medications are called "Antianxiety and sedative-hypnotic agents" (28). Introduced nearly 30 years ago, the benzodiazepines were identified as having few drawbacks then other medications and were safer in combination with other agents. Today, these medications are still the most widely prescribed in terms of reducing anxiety. SSRI's such as zoloft, paxil, lexapro and luvox are also prescribed for anxiety. These medications work by blocking the re-uptake of serotonin into the neuron, thus increasing serotonin levels. Consultation with a knowledgeable psychiatrist would be advised if you believe that your patient might need medication to monitor her moods, thoughts or emotions. If you are unclear about the current medication regiment your patient is taking or have questions, this type of consultation is recommended.

COMPLEMENTARY AND
ALTERNATIVE MEDICINE (CAM)

CAM refers to the different mind/body strategies that are not generally practiced in western medicine. CAM is an umbrella term that covers a variety of treatment strategies such as Theta Healing , acupuncture, herbs, minerals, homeopathy, vitamins, Reiki, as well as many others. These treatments can be useful to the dietitian because they are often readily available, easily accessible, and can be learned fairly quickly. More information on these can be found in Chapter 5.

ADDITIONAL STRATEGIES FOR THE DIETITIAN
WORKING WITH WOMEN DIAGNOSED WITH PCOS

Because of the nature of PCOS, the process of weight loss will not be similar to a client with no endocrine issues. Therefore, to avoid adding additional stress and disappointment to your client, being mindful of the PCOS diagnosis would be advantageous. Consideration should be made to the weight loss goal with intermediary short-term goals. Creating goals that are not geared around weight may be most beneficial. If weight goals are desired, try setting a goal where your client will maintain a current weight, rather than losing weight. You may want to approach your client with the goal of gaining less weight than usual. Ideally, being creative and thinking "outside the box" with these clients will serve you best. A collaborative approach, or coming to goals together as a team, might assist this patient in not only creating goals that are realistic, but also goals that will be ascertained.

Additional goals for women with PCOS might be following a healthy eating regiment, meeting exercise quotas, using coping skills with urges, practicing mindful eating, or successful healthy dining-out. Food logs for these patients might need to include information other then just the type and quantity of food consumed. Other information to be logged might be times of meals, places of meal consumption, or situations/feelings that occur surrounding food consumption.

As the dietitian, you can also set up small rewards that your clients can earn by meeting their goals. For instance, you may decide to have a weekly drawing for a gift certificate for a spa treatment or something equally desirable for which your clients can be eligible for if they have met their weekly goal. Remember to stress with your PCOS clients that the goal is healthy choices rather than "healthy weight."

CHAPTER SUMMARY

- **Women with PCOS may have a greater likelihood of facing mental health issues such as poor body image, low self-esteem, stress, anxiety, depression, and bipolar disorder than other women.**
- **Although there has been a great deal of research done on the psychological impact of the individual symptoms of PCOS, there is still a paucity of research on evaluating the mental health status of women with PCOS.**
- **There are different treatment strategies available for women with PCOS that include prescription medication, and psychotherapy and complementary and alternative medicines.**
- **Dietitians can use different strategies to help set appropriate goals for women diagnosed with PCOS to empower her to succeed with a healthy lifestyle.**

REFERENCES

1. Himelein M.J., Thatcher S.S. Depression and body image among women with polycystic ovary syndrome. *Journal of Health Psychology.* 2006;11(4):613-25.

2. Himelein M.J., Thatcher, S.S. Polycystic ovary syndrome and mental health: A Review. *Obstetrical and Gynecological Survey.* 2006;61(11):723-732.

3. American Psychological Association. Americans engage in unhealthy behaviors to manage stress. February 2003. Retrieved from http://apahelpcenter.mediaroom.com/index. php?s=press_releases&item=23

4. Rutledge, T, Linden W. To Eat or Not to Eat: Affective and Physiological Mechanisms in the Stress–Eating Relationship. *Journal of Behavioral Medicine.* 1998;21(3):221-240.

5. Epel E, Lapidus R., McEwen B, Brownell K. Stress may add bite to appetite in women: a laboratory study of stress-induced cortisol and eating behavior. *Psychoneuroendocrinology,* 2001;26(1):37-49.

6. Lipton M.G., Sherr L, Elford J, Rustin M.H.A., Clayton W.J. Women living with facial hair: The psychological and behavioral burden. *Journal of Psychosomatic Research. 2006; 61*:161-168.

7. Connolly KJ, Edelmann RJ, Cooke ID, Robson J. The impact of infertility on psychological functioning. *Journal of Psychosomatic Research.* 1992; 36(5):459-68.

8. Trent M.E, Rich M., Austin S.B, et al. Fertility concerns and sexual behavior in adolescent girls with polycystic ovary syndrome. *Journal of Pediatric Adolescent Gynecology.* 2003;16:33-37.

9. Elsenbruch S, Hahn S, Kowalsky D, Offner A.H, Schedlowski M, Mann K, Janssen O.E. Quality of life, psychosocial well-being, and sexual satisfaction in women with polycystic ovary syndrome. *The Journal of Clinical Endocrinology and Metabolism.* 2003;88:5801-5807.

10. Conaglen H.M, Conaglen JV. Sexual desire in women presenting for antiandrogen therapy. *Journal of Sexual and Marital Therapy.* 2003;29:255-267.

11. Homberg R. The Management of Infertility Associated With Polycystic Ovary Syndrome. *Reproductive Biology and Endocrinology. 2003: V.*

12. Chambless D.L, Baker M.J, Baucom D.H, Beutler L.D, Calhoun K.S,

Critis-Cristoph P et al. Update on empirically validated therapies II. *The Clinical Psychologist.1998;51*(1):3-16.

13. Woody S.R., Weisz J., McLean C. Empirically supported treatments: 10 Years later. *The Clinical Psychologist. 2005;* 58(4):5-11.

14. American Psychological Association Diagnostic and statistical manual of mental disorders, 4th ed. Washington DC: American Psychological Association, 2000.

15. Spitzer, R.L., Devlin, M., Walsh. B.T., Hasin, D et al. Binge eating disorder: A multisite field trial of the diagnostic criteria. *International Journal of Eating Disorders.* 1992;11(3):191-203.

16. Rasgon, N.L., Rao, R.C., Hwang, S., Altshuler, L.L., Elman, S., Zuckerbrow-Miller, J, Korenman, S.G. Depression in women with polycystic ovary syndrome: clinical and biochemical correlates. *Journal of Affective Disorders.* 2003;74:299-304.

17. Rasgon, N.L., Reynolds, M.F., Elman, S., Saad, M., Frye, M.A., Bauer, M., Altshuler, L.L. Longitudinal evaluation of reproductive function in women treated for bipolar disorder. *Journal of Affective Disorders.* 2005;89:217-225.

18. Clausen, J.O., Borch-Johnsen, K., Ibsen, H., Bergman, R.N., Hougaard, P et al. Insulin sensitivity index, acute insulin response, and glucose effectiveness in a population-based sample of 380 young healthy Caucasians. Analysis of the impact of gender, body fat, physical fitness, and lifestyle factors. Journal of Clinical Investigation. 1996;98,:1195–1209.

19. Brown, A.J. Depression and insulin resistance: Applications to polycystic ovary syndrome. *Clinical Obstetrics and Gynecology.* 2004;47(3):592-596.

20. Okamura F, Tashiro A, Utumi A, et al. Insulin resistance in patients with depression and its changes during the clinical course of depression: minimal model analysis. *Metabolism.* 2000; 49:1255-1260.

21. Amsterdam, J.D., Shults, J., Rutherford, N., Schwartz, S. (2006). Safety and efficacy of s-citalopram in patients with co-morbid major depression and diabetes mellitus. *Neuropsychobiology,* 54(4), 208-14.

22. Keegan A., Liao LM, Boyle, M. 'Hirsutism': a psychological analysis. *Journal of Health Psychology.* 2003; 8:327-345.

23. Weiner, C.L., Primeau, M., Ehrmann, D.A.. Androgens and mood dysfunction in women: comparison of women with polycystic

ovarian syndrome to healthy controls. *Psychosomatic Medicine.* 2004;66:356-362.

24.   Joffe H., Kim D., Foris J.M., Baldassano C.F., Gyulai L., Hwang C.H., et al. Menstrual dysfunction prior to onset of psychiatric illness is reported more commonly by women with bipolar disorder than by with unipolar depression and healthy controls. *Journal of Clinical Psychiatry.* 2006;67(2):297-304.

25.   Klipstein K., Goldberg J. Screening for bipolar disorder in women with polycystic ovary syndrome: A pilot study. *Journal of Affective Disorders.* 2006;97:205–209.

26.   Beck A.T, Emery G. Anxiety disorders and Phobias: A Cognitive Perspective. Basic Books, 1985.

27.   Telch C.F., Agras W.S., Linehan M.M. Dialectical behavior therapy for binge eating disorder. *Journal of Consulting and Clinical Psychology. 2001;69:*1060-1065.

28.   Janicak P.G, Davis J.M, Preshkorn S.H., Ayd F.J. *Principles and Practice of Psychopharacotherapy.* Lippincott Williams & Wilkins; Philadelphia 1997.

CHAPTER 3

DIETARY STRATEGIES AND LIFESTYLE MODIFICATION

MUCH CONFUSION EXISTS ABOUT the proper dietary approaches women with PCOS should implement to improve their symptoms and lab parameters, lose weight, regulate their menstrual function, and decrease risk for chronic diseases. There is consensus that these women must manage their insulin resistance and further weight gain. Blood pressure and lipid levels often need to be decreased, especially triglycerides (these tend to become elevated when insulin levels are high) to reduce the risk of cardiovascular disease. Many women will seek the advice of a dietitian primarily to lose weight and improve dermatological symptoms. In addition, weight loss helps to regulate menstrual cycles and improve fertility. All of these situations can be improved with proper dietary and lifestyle changes, demonstrating that medical nutrition therapy (MNT) interventions play a crucial part in the physical and emotional health of PCOS women.

The majority of patients I have treated with PCOS are focused on weight loss, as they want to lose the central weight that was gained so rapidly and uncontrollably. Most of them are unhappy, even hating their bodies at times for having PCOS and being so different from other women. Most have been spent their lives battling their weight with limited success at weight loss. It is common for some to have the extreme belief that they need to limit their carbohydrate intake as much as possible in order to lose weight. Unfortunately, this leads to an unhealthy preoccupation with food that often comes with dieting. As discussed in Chapter 8, it is very common for many women with PCOS to develop distorted eating patterns or full-blown eating disorders. Keep in mind that the majority of women with PCOS have struggled with their weight for most of their lives, probably due to the hormonal influence of years of elevated insulin and testosterone levels; they are almost accustomed to the dieting cycle and body loathing.

Most of the low carbohydrate advice patients acquire comes primarily from the internet or from misinformed health care providers who believe that the best treatment for women with PCOS is to eat a very low carbohydrate diet in order to reduce elevated insulin levels. In fact, it is very common for physicians to tell their PCOS patients to follow diets such as Sugar Busters or the Atkins Diet to lose weight. However, as this chapter examines the most recent studies on diet composition and PCOS, we see that this does not have to be the case. Before the mid 1990s there was limited research regarding diet composition and PCOS. Perhaps this is because PCOS was regarded as a reproductive disorder, not as an endocrine one. In fact, to date only 3 articles and no scientific studies have ever been published in the *Journal of The American Dietetic Association* on PCOS (1-3), the primary source where dietitians obtain their evidence base regarding MNT. Additionally, much of the research presented on PCOS comes from observational studies, case studies, and clinical experience due to the lack of established MNT recommendations. It is no surprise that dietitians may be unaware of an appropriate dietary approach. The purpose of this chapter is to examine the effects of different diet compositions on PCOS and reach a conclusion as to what diet modalities and lifestyle modifications benefit women with PCOS the most. The following chapter will discuss how dietitians can implement recommended diet strategies for PCOS with their patients.

THE IMPORTANCE OF DIET AND LIFESTYLE MANAGEMENT IN THE TREATMENT OF POLYCYSTIC OVARY SYNDROME

The prevalence of impaired glucose tolerance (IGT) is 31 to 35% in women with PCOS as well as a 7.5 to 10% prevalence of type 2 diabetes mellitus (T2DM) (4,5). With insulin resistance and hyperinsulinemia now recognized as the underlying factors in the pathogenesis of PCOS, it is evident that lowering insulin levels and improving insulin sensitivity are the key strategies in managing the syndrome and preventing the onset of other clinical manifestations such as hyperlipidemia and the metabolic syndrome (MBS). Elevated insulin appears to be the catalyst leading to the production of elevated androgens in women with PCOS (6). Treatment aimed to reduce insulin levels will lower androgen levels and improve metabolic and reproductive symptoms, as well as lower health risks for T2DM and heart disease (6). What has remained questionable until recently is, "what is the best dietary treatment approach to do this?"

Several studies have shown beneficial effects of the insulin sensitizer metformin (glucophage®, Bristol-Myers Squibb Co.) in improving all PCOS symptoms (7-9). However, recent evidence also suggests that diet and lifestyle may be just as effective if not *more* effective in managing PCOS (10-15). Because women with PCOS experience a high degree of insulin resistance and IGT that puts them at an increased risk for T2DM, we can apply information obtained from The Diabetes Prevention Program (DPP) to the treatment of PCOS. In this National Institute of Health sponsored study involving 2,345 overweight and obese individuals, researchers found that lifestyle modification (diet and exercise) achieved a 58% reduction in risk of progression from IGT to T2DM and reduced incidence of MBS by 41%. The lifestyle intervention group had a 31% greater reduction in risk for diabetes than from metformin alone (16). The average weight loss was a modest 6%.

Furthermore, in a study on the effects of exercise and nutritional counseling on women with PCOS, Bruner et al found that nutritional counseling, with or without exercise, decreased insulin levels and improved both metabolic and reproductive abnormalities associated with PCOS (17). This emphasizes the need to promote lifestyle modification techniques as the primary treatment for PCOS in conjunction with pharmacological interventions. Obviously, early detection and intervention of IGT in women with PCOS is crucial. For this reason, the American Association of Clinical Endocrinologists and American College of Endocrinology have recommended screening for diabetes with an oral glucose tolerance test (OGTT) by the age of 30, for all patients with PCOS (18). Assessing fasting insulin levels should also be part of the OGTT. It is important to note that it is common for women with PCOS to have normal fasting glucose readings despite having elevated insulin levels (9,14).

Women with PCOS are at a higher risk than other women for the development of cardiovascular disease due to the increased prevalence of hypertension, dyslipidemia (low high-density lipoprotein cholesterol (HDL), elevated low-density lipoprotein cholesterol (LDL) and high triglycerides), C-reactive protein (CRP), atherosclerotic disease and endothelial dysfunction (9,6). It is estimated that 70% of women with PCOS show low levels of HDL and elevated LDL levels (19). Not surprisingly, women with PCOS also have high rates of MBS with a prevalence of 43% (20). This is a 2-fold higher than the age-adjusted prevalence rate of 24% in women nationally, based on women in the NHANES III survey (21). In contrast to normal women, insulin resistance in PCOS appears to be the main cause of abnormal lipids, blood pressure, and androgens (6). Studies conducted with metformin demonstrate a significant change in dyslipidemia in women with PCOS (20-22). Diet modification and exercise can certainly have a positive effect on cardiovascular risk factors. Metformin combined with diet has been shown to improve many features of MBS including reducing serum triglycerides, total and LDL cholesterol, and blood pressure (20).

Lifestyle interventions involving behavioral, dietary, and exercise management should be the primary focus of treatment for women with PCOS. Pharmacological treatment, including the use of insulin-sensitizing agents, should be used as a secondary strategy. MNT therefore plays an integral role in preventing and treating the clinical manifestations associated with PCOS; it reinforces the need for adequate knowledge and training among dietetic professionals in working with the PCOS population.

DO WOMEN WITH PCOS REALLY EAT MORE?

Before I was diagnosed with PCOS the main indicator that I knew something was not right with my body was a period when I consistently gained weight each month without any changes to my eating or exercise routine. The majority of the weight gain centered in my mid-section. In addition, I found that despite managing my caloric intake and physical activity patterns, I was not able to lose weight. I have heard this from many of my PCOS clients, including some who are athletes, exercise physiologists, or even personal trainers; all reported gaining weight without changes to diet or exercise, and not being able to lose it.

As dietitians, we are accustomed to hearing patients tell us that they can't lose weight even though they are exercising and limiting their caloric intake. We know that many may be eating more than they think and under reporting their intake. However, in the case of PCOS when insulin levels are elevated, it causes the body to store fat very easily and prevents the breakdown of fat (lipolysis). It is theorized that high insulin levels act as an appetite stimulant that cause individuals to crave food more, especially refined or high glycemic-index (GI) carbohydrate foods (12,14,23). The need for more carbohydrates may even occur shortly after eating a large meal. For example, many patients report intense carbohydrate cravings soon after eating dinner, even though they are not hungry. One of the questions I always ask any of my clients during the nutrition assessment, regardless of the reason why they came to see me is "what types of foods do you crave?" Usually the clients with PCOS will respond by saying that the food they mostly crave is carbohydrate-rich.

Recently, researchers looked at the diet composition of 30 PCOS women versus non-PCOS women of the same BMI, race, and age group (24). Although they found that the women with PCOS ate essentially the same diet in regards to total energy and macronutrient intake, women with PCOS consumed a slightly higher amount of total fat and a greater quantity of high GI foods. The women with PCOS also had elevated insulin levels (24). This study concluded that those with PCOS do not necessarily eat more food but may eat a diet composed of higher amounts of simple carbohydrates (probably related to their elevated insulin levels) and higher amounts of fat.

Appetite regulation is another difference between women with PCOS and non-PCOS women in regards to weight management. Leptin, ghrelin and cholecystokinin (CCK) levels have all been found to be dysfunctional in PCOS (25,26). CCK, a hormone derived from the small intestine, is released postprandially in response to protein and fat in the duodenum; it inhibits gastric emptying and signals satiety. When matched with controls, overweight women with PCOS were found to have reduced postprandial CCK response (25). While it is not known why women with PCOS have impaired CCK secretion following meals, it has been suggested that they may have delayed gastric emptying (25).

Fasting levels of ghrelin, the stomach-derived hormone that is secreted preprandially to signal hunger, has also been found to be impaired in lean and obese women with PCOS compared to weight matched non-PCOS women (27,28). In one study, overweight subjects with PCOS were less satiated and hungrier after test meals than over-weight subjects without PCOS (28).

In addition, it has been speculated that leptin, which is involved in energy balance and reproduction, may be implicated in the pathophys-iology of PCOS (26). A positive correlation exists between leptin and BMI and between leptin and testosterone in women with PCOS (29). Decreased leptin function may stimulate feeding in PCOS women, resulting in increased food intake and difficulties managing weight (30). In addition, having impaired levels of CCK and ghrelin could also explain why PCOS women are resistant to weight loss as appetite signals are compromised, making them hungrier and wanting to eat more.

The main reason why PCOS women tend to be heavier is mostly due to elevated androgen and insulin levels, especially if the weight is primarily in the central part of the body. As you continue to treat more women with PCOS, you will start to become familiar with the android distribution shape these women have and will be able to start recognizing it among clients whom you suspect may have PCOS or elevated insulin levels. Early on in my work with PCOS I was amazed when I attended my first Polycystic Ovary Association symposium. All around were hundreds of women who looked so much alike, all of whom had excess weight around their waist even though the rest of their body was more slender. You may even start to notice women outside of your office, in public places, like at the supermarket checkout counter or at the airport whom you suspect may have PCOS because of their unique shape and appearance. I often have to bite my lip to resist being too intrusive by suggesting the possibility of PCOS to some strangers who I suspect have it!

DOES THE AMERICAN DIET CAUSE PCOS?

Even though there appears to be a strong genetic component to PCOS with many women having a mother, sister, or grandmother with the syndrome, it has also been proposed that perhaps diet may contribute to its development. When PCOS was first discovered in 1935 it was seen primarily as a reproductive disorder. However, as it is estimated that 60-80% of women with PCOS in the United States are insulin resistant with compensatory hyperinsulinemia (31), PCOS is now mostly seen as an endocrine disorder. Since the majority of women with PCOS are obese, it has lead some to speculate that obesity or lifestyle also may lead to the development of the syndrome. A linear correlation between BMI and insulin resistance has been documented showing that heavier women with PCOS who have more abdominal fat have greater amounts of insulin resistance than thinner women with PCOS (32).

Excessive carbohydrate consumption is associated with the development of MBS (10). When the diet composition of PCOS versus non-PCOS matched controls was analyzed, researchers discovered that the most common high GI foods consumed among the PCOS women were white bread (24). This includes hamburger and hot dog rolls and potatoes, all of which are commonly found in American's diets. Although the PCOS women consumed a greater intake of high GI foods, total carbohydrate intake was the same between the matched PCOS and non-PCOS women. This led the researchers to suggest that the quality of carbohydrate, in addition to a lifestyle of a higher fast food consumption (which is known to be high in white bread and saturated fat and low in fiber) may be conducive to the development of the syndrome (24).

An association also exists between a high saturated fat intake and reduced insulin sensitivity as well as an increased risk of developing T2DM (15). Interestingly, when the diet composition of PCOS women in the United States were compared to those in Italy, caloric intake was similar but women in the U.S. consumed more saturated fat. Women in the U.S. also showed a higher BMI (33). Theoretically, it could be possible for some women to develop insulin resistance and PCOS from their eating style, especially because so many Americans consume fast food and lead a sedentary lifestyle. Of course, this is one theory and much more research is needed in this area. Presently, the majority of women who have PCOS usually do have a first-degree relative with the syndrome, suggesting more genetic tendency than lifestyle.

HIGH PROTEIN DIETS AND PCOS

A high protein and low-carbohydrate (<100 grams/day or < 30% total calories) diet has been traditionally thought to aid in weight loss and improve metabolic and reproductive dysfunction in PCOS (11,12,34). Perhaps due to the satiating effect of protein in preventing or decreasing hunger as compared to carbohydrate or fat, or improving insulin sensitivity through the maintenance of lean body mass with weight loss, high protein/low carbohydrate diets have been seen as the premier dietary treatment for PCOS (34). However, contrary to public belief, there is little evidence to suggest the benefits of high protein diets on lowering insulin levels and improving insulin resistance or other parameters in PCOS (34-36). While protein foods do not cause the same degree of insulin release in the body that carbohydrates do, they still do elicit a response, of what effect is still unknown (15,34). Yet, many health professionals and consumers believe that limiting carbohydrates is the only way to reduce insulin levels, lose weight and improve PCOS symptoms. Little do they know that high protein diets may actually make insulin resistance worse and impair glucose metabolism, plus contribute to weight gain and hypertension. This can put women with PCOS at a higher risk for developing heart disease and T2DM as these diets are typically higher in saturated fat and cholesterol and lower in fruits, vegetables, and whole grains as recommended by national dietary guidelines.

Several studies examined the role of diet composition and its effect in treating women with PCOS. In one study, 28 overweight or obese women with PCOS were chosen to follow either a high-protein or low-protein diet of the same caloric content (1400 calories) for 3 months (34). Half of the women followed a high-protein diet composed of 40% carbohydrates, 30% protein, and 30% fat. The other half followed a low-protein diet composed of 55% carbohydrate, 15% protein, 30% fat. Both groups showed similar results regardless of diet composition in lowering of insulin and testosterone levels, improving sex-hormone binding globulin (SHBG), and improving menstrual function. Additionally, there was no significant difference in weight loss between the two groups (34).

Other studies of shorter duration and smaller sample size used the same study design to compare high versus low protein diets with a similar diet composition (35,24). They confirmed the same results: a high protein diet does not differ from that of a low protein diet in improving metabolic and reproductive parameters in PCOS women. Furthermore, in both studies, weight loss was not significantly different between the two diet composition groups. These studies show that energy restricted diets are beneficial at producing weight loss in women with PCOS, as well as improving insulin sensitivity, testosterone, SHBG, and menstrual function. However, a high protein diet does not improve these parameters any more than a diet of lower protein or higher carbohydrate content. Thus, there is no reason for women with PCOS to severely limit their carbohydrate intake and follow a high protein diet for weight loss for improvement of their symptoms.

As many dietitians know, there are many health risks associated with high protein diets. Usually high protein diets are accompanied by foods high in saturated fat and cholesterol (i.e. cheeses, meats, eggs) which could worsen lipid levels and put women with PCOS at an even higher risk for cardiovascular disease. High protein diets can lead to osteoporosis and kidney stones (12). They can also contribute to hypertension and cancer through the avoidance of important vitamins, minerals, fiber, and antioxidants found in fruits, vegetables, and whole grains. Additionally, most people are not able to follow a high-protein, low-carbohydrate diet for very long. They may experience some weight loss from these types of diets due to energy restriction and initial body water loss, however, most will find them too difficult to adhere to over time. This often leads to overeating and weight gain once they do start to introduce carbohydrates back into the diet, worsening lab parameters. Self-esteem is affected and may cause individuals to have negative attitudes toward food and their bodies. Women with PCOS may have a particularly harder time following these types of diets which limit carbohydrates long-term; they may have more hypoglycemic episodes and/or crave carbohydrates more than most people. If these women do attempt these diets (and most of them do), they often are left with added feelings of shame, hopelessness, and failure if they cannot maintain them long-term.

VERY LOW-CALORIE DIETS AND PCOS

Tolino et al examined the effect of long-term caloric restriction on both clinical and biochemical abnormalities in 114 obese women with PCOS (37). The subjects followed a strict, low calorie diet of 500 calories/day for 4 weeks followed by 1,000 calories/day for 7 months. Fifty-four percent of the women lost more than 5% of body weight, while 11.8% remained at pretreatment weight despite the severely limited caloric amount for the obese women, demonstrating the difficulty women with PCOS have losing weight. Both groups showed improvements in testosterone levels. Those who lost weight had significant improvements in blood levels of insulin and 81.8% showed improvement in reproductive function despite no significant changes in LH or follicle-stimulating hormone (FSH) levels (37).

Another study compared the effects of meal replacements on short-term weight loss, followed by dietary macronutrient restriction for six months (38). Forty-three overweight women with PCOS ate meal replacements for two meals per day for 8 weeks, then half of the subjects followed either a low carbohydrate (<120 grams/day) diet or a low fat (< 50 grams/day) diet for 24 weeks. A reduction in weight (6%) and waist circumference (6 cm) occurred, as well as improvements in fasting insulin, testosterone and free androgen index (38). Meal replacements appear to be an effective strategy for short-term weight loss, however, no significant difference was found with regards to diet composition among the 2 groups (38). In general, severe caloric restriction can cause short-term weight loss and improve PCOS parameters. However, long-term adherence to these diets is extremely difficult. Those that experience dietary relapse will often regain weight. Once weight is regained, the manifestations of PCOS and the associated long-term morbidity and mortality risks will probably also return (13). Instructing clients to follow such diets is therefore ineffective and will only contribute to worsening of self-esteem, eating habits, and health. Treatment should therefore emphasize a combination of diet modification, physical activity, and behavior change.

LOW-FAT DIETS FOR WOMEN WITH PCOS

Traditionally, low-fat diets were advised for weight loss, especially in improving MBS (10). However, according to Willet (39), short-term trials of low fat diets resulted in minimal changes in body weight and that long-term trials (greater than 1 year) also showed little or no weight loss. Recent research implies that a higher carbohydrate intake, particularly from refined carbohydrates, combined with a low-fat diet can actually make MBS worse; it can exaggerate postprandial glycemia and increase obesity (23). In fact, focusing on low-fat, high GI diets can be problematic as they can increase triglyceride levels and decrease HDL concentrations, and worsen blood pressure (10,12). Low-fat recommendations can actually promote higher consumption of refined carbohydrates, especially because manufacturers tend to add sugar to reduced fat products. Too little fat in the diet can also contribute to hunger, overeating, and weight gain as fat contributes to satiety.

THE GLYCEMIC INDEX DIET
FOR WOMEN WITH PCOS

Like high protein diets, the GI diet has also risen in popularity among women with PCOS to help manage insulin levels and lose weight, but this approach has not yet been studied in the PCOS population. The GI diet was originally developed by researchers in Toronto in 1981. The premise of the diet is based on the quality of carbohydrate and its effect on the body's postprandial blood glucose. The GI approach ranks foods numerically on their effect on blood sugar levels 2-3 hours after eating. Foods with a high GI are proposed to break down quickly during digestion, causing a quick release of glucose into the bloodstream. In contrast, low GI foods either contain carbohydrates that break down more slowly, or fiber that slows absorption of carbohydrates resulting in a more gradual release of glucose into the bloodstream.

The GI diet was developed in a laboratory by giving test subjects, with or without diabetes, 50 grams of an "available" carbohydrate food (without factoring grams of fiber) under fasting conditions to see what degree their blood sugar would rise. They then compared the response of the selected food to a reference food containing the same amount of carbohydrate (usually glucose or table sugar) and converted it into a numeric ranking system. For example, glucose has a GI of 100, whereas carrots have a GI of 47. A listing of GI foods can easily be found by searching on the internet. Generally, the GI ranges are as follows:

Low GI = < 55
Medium GI = 56-69
High GI = > 70

The concept is for individuals to choose foods that have the lowest GI values in order to have less of a rise in postprandial glucose after eating, thus requiring less insulin to regulate blood sugar. Not surprisingly, most of the foods with a low GI contain a significant amount of fiber which causes food to be digested and absorbed more slowly. Fiber produces a feeling of fullness, and is an added benefit for those trying to lose weight and control insulin and/or glucose levels.

However, the GI focuses on the quality of carbohydrate and not the *quantity*. To determine the degree of rise in blood sugar per portion size, researchers have developed the glycemic load (GL). The GL is calculated by multiplying the GI of a food by the amount of carbohydrate per serving and dividing by 100 and provides a better estimate of quantity and quality of carbohydrate. Like the GI, there are also ranges classifying GL values:

Low GI = $\leq$ 10
Medium GI = 11-19
High GI = $\geq$ 20

For example, watermelon has a GI of 72 (high) and 6 grams of carbohydrate (not counting fiber grams) per serving and has a low GL, (72 x 6)/100 = 4.32. Therefore, the GI is more useful in comparing foods but the GL is useful when you need to know the content per serving.

While there are numerous benefits to consuming foods with a low GI and GL, the GI diet itself has many disadvantages. Many critics suggest that the foods selected and tested were studied under artificial conditions in the laboratory and don't reflect the mixed meals that more accurately represent what the pubic really eats. Indeed, many factors can influence postprandial blood sugar levels including the shelf life of the food, cooking and processing methods as well as the fat, protein, and fiber content of the food. Additionally, the glucose response to a particular food is individual. It is also nearly impossible for consumers to memorize the GI of individual foods. The bottom line is that the GI diet itself is impractical, since too many variables exist that can affect a GI rating. Therefore, I don't encourage or instruct PCOS clients to follow the GI diet consisting of numerical rankings. Instead, I advise them to eat foods that are of 'low GI' -that is high fiber, and minimally processed whole grain foods which have been shown to improve insulin sensitivity, decrease cardiovascular risk, and aid in weight loss.

BENEFITS OF CONSUMING LOW GLYCEMIC INDEX DIETS FOR PCOS

Presently, there is conflicting evidence about the weight loss effects of low GI diets (40). In one study, subjects did not show a weight loss at one year when educated on the GI diet (41). However, effects of low GI diets may depend on the population studied (40). In one study, overweight men and women with normal glucose tolerance followed low and high GL diets for 6 months. Those with high insulin secretion 30 minutes after an oral glucose load lost more weight than those with lower insulin secretion (42). This suggests that individuals with elevated insulin levels respond more favorably to modifications in carbohydrate content.

A study examined the relationship between a diet consistent with the 2005 Dietary Guidelines for Americans and measures of insulin resistance in the Framingham Heart Study Offspring Cohort. An association existed mainly among women in the study, with those scoring the highest for meeting the Dietary Guidelines having the lowest measures of insulin resistance (43). This led the researchers to speculate that a diet consistent with the 2005 Dietary Guidelines that includes whole grains, fruits, and vegetables may be an effective way to limit insulin resistance in women.

Dietary GI may relate to insulin sensitivity for many reasons. One main reason could be that high GI foods elicit a rapid rise in blood glucose and therefore a rapid release of insulin, resulting in hypoglycemia (reactive hypoglycemia). Many women with PCOS exhibit frequent bouts of hypoglycemia. Conversely, low GI foods cause a reduced and prolonged postprandial insulin release and tend to prevent hypoglycemia (12).

Findings of a larger and longer study (18 months) published in the *Journal of the American Medical Association* showed more promising results regarding the effects of a low GI diet versus a low-fat diet in regards to weight loss (44). In this study, researchers measured the insulin levels of 73 obese adults (ages 18-35) without diabetes, using a 75 gram glucose tolerance test. One group was instructed to reduce carbohydrate intake to a maximum of 40% of calories and to consume only low GI foods. A second group was able to eat a variety of carbohydrate-containing foods (~55%) but had to limit fat intake to 20% of calories. Both groups reduced their calories by about 400 calories/day (44).

After following the diets for 18 months, subjects with the highest insulin spikes at the beginning of the study lost a significant amount of weight (13 lbs. on average) following the low GI diet while those that followed the low-fat diet lost just an average of 3 lbs. Those with low insulin levels at the start of the study also only lost an average of 3 lbs. regardless of what diet they followed (44). In addition, the low GI diet was associated with greater improvements in HDL, LDL, and triglyceride levels than the low-fat diet.

The energy balance equation, in which calories consumed must equal those expended, does not appear to be applicable to individuals with elevated insulin. This suggests that changes in diet composition by eating a lower GI diet must occur in conjunction with a caloric restricted diet to achieve significant weight loss. These results are encouraging to women with PCOS who have elevated insulin levels and further reinforce the difficulties these women have in losing weight.

Another study suggests that changes in dietary GL is more effective in weight loss among women than men. When four reduced-calorie (1400 calorie) diets of varying GL where compared, women in the two reduced GI diets had an 80% greater fat loss than men when compared to low-fat diets (23).

A higher intake of fiber from whole grains has been shown to decrease the risk of developing T2DM. In the Nurses Health Study, an inverse relationship was found between cereal fiber intake and a low GI diet and the risk of T2DM (45). Both normal and diabetic subjects had lower blood glucose levels and decreased insulin secretion in response to a low GI diet containing pumpernickel bread with intact whole grains, bulgur, pasta and legumes in comparison to a high GI diet. Researchers suggest that whole grains can slow the digestion and absorption of carbohydrates, thus decreasing postprandial glucose and insulin response (46).

Consuming a low GI diet may also be favorable with PCOS in regards to cardiovascular health. Ludwig reported on 13 studies examining the effects of different GI diets with similar diet composition on serum lipids in individuals with hyperlipidemia and diabetes (47). The majority of the studies demonstrated that a low GI diet can decrease triglycerides, LDL and total/HDL cholesterol ratio (47). Consumption of whole grains has also been linked to reducing the risk of CHD. Van Dam et al report that diets consisting of refined carbohydrates (high GI) that do not include low GI foods are associated with higher serum cholesterol levels (48), findings that other studies support (23,47). In the Framingham Offspring study, individuals with the highest quartile of GI foods had higher rates of MBS and insulin resistance when compared with those who consumed the lowest quartile of GI foods (49).

The Dietary Approaches to Stop Hypertension (DASH) study further exemplifies the benefits of consuming a low GI diet. Participants in the DASH study showed significant improvements in lipids and blood pressure despite a relatively high (57%) carbohydrate intake consisting of high amounts of fruits, vegetables, whole grain foods and low-fat dairy products (50). When the DASH diet was implemented in the PREMIER Interventions on Insulin Sensitivity study, a greater improvement in insulin sensitivity was found with the DASH diet than without it (51). Dietary composition of the DASH diet also reduced components of MBS (10), further supporting the benefits of a lower GI eating plan for women with PCOS.

All of this evidence suggests that both the type and amount of carbohydrate in the diet are important. Moderate amounts of carbohydrates, if in the low GI form, can actually be beneficial to the treatment of PCOS; it can improve insulin sensitivity, glucose tolerance, hyperlipidemia, and overall MBS. Low GI foods contain more fiber and take longer to chew, which tends to increase satiety, reduce hunger, and lower subsequent voluntary food intake. In contrast, high GI foods have been known to stimulate appetite leading to greater food intake (15). Therefore, carbohydrates do not need to be avoided in the PCOS diet, but the type and quantity have to be modified for optimal results. A diet low in saturated fat and high in fiber from whole grain foods can improve both short and long-term symptoms of PCOS, as well as decrease risk of chronic diseases associated with insulin resistance.

THE ROLE OF DIETARY FAT

Like carbohydrates, it appears that both the type (saturated, polyunsaturated (PUFA), monounsaturated (MUFA), and *trans* fat) and amount of fat are important. A high intake of saturated and *trans* fatty acids has been found to cause dyslipidemia and hyperinsulinemia, increasing the risk for diabetes and MBS. A large, prospective study conducted on more than 80,000 women enrolled in the Nurses' Health Study found that substituting mono and polyunsaturated fats for just 5% of saturated fat calories reduced the risk of coronary heart disease in women by 42% (52). Researchers from this study also suggest that replacing saturated fats with unsaturated fats is more effective in preventing coronary heart disease than decreasing overall fat intake (52). Consumption of omega-3 fatty acids has been demonstrated to be beneficial in decreasing insulin resistance (53). Its use is also beneficial to those with MBS and T2DM and subsequently women with PCOS, since they have the ability to reduce triglycerides and LDL concentrations, increase HDL concentrations, lower blood pressure and glucose levels, and improve insulin sensitivity (10,54).

Despite the possible benefits of a higher unsaturated fat diet in improving insulin resistance, a major concern of these diets is the possibility of weight gain due to the high caloric content of dietary fat. Current NCEP ATP III guidelines suggest total fat should range between 25-35%, while limiting saturated fat to less than 7%. PUFA should be up to 10% and MUFA up to 20% of total calories (55). Women with PCOS will need slightly greater amounts of total fat coming from MUFA and PUFA sources to substitute for the reduction in carbohydrate intake.

WEIGHT LOSS AND PCOS

From personal experience and from the patients that I have worked with, I can tell you that weight loss is very difficult for women with PCOS to achieve. Is it possible for PCOS women to lose weight? Absolutely, but it is a very slow process and can be frustrating, especially to the patient who expects immediate results. Even with sustained changes to diet and activity, some women will still not be able to lose significant amounts of weight. Sometimes it seems that in order to see some weight loss occur in PCOS women, insulin levels must come down at least somewhat. This could take months, and it requires regular monitoring of fasting insulin levels (every 3 months or so) to see if changes in diet, activity, or medication are necessary.

One study that looked at treatment of PCOS with metformin (850 mg/twice daily) for 6 months, found that metformin, when added to a hypocaloric diet, results in a greater reduction of body weight and abdominal fat, as well as insulin, testosterone, and leptin levels in comparison to placebo (8). Many patients who take metformin are under the impression (again from misinformed health care providers or from the internet) that they will automatically lose weight from the medication. This is not necessarily the case. Some women will lose weight, usually not much, when they first start taking metformin. However, this could be due to lack of interest in food, reduced cravings, diarrhea (the main side effect), or it could be due to a placebo effect. Other individuals may not experience any weight loss from metformin at all, but instead find it will at least aid in preventing further weight gain. I have found that in almost all patients who start taking metformin that they are able to stop gaining weight. Nonetheless, metformin should not be viewed as a weight loss drug. Patients who are taking metformin or who are about to start taking it need to be educated that changes in eating and activity must also occur in order to achieve weight loss. For some women, metformin may not be effective in decreasing insulin levels on its own and may require the addition of other insulin-sensitizing drugs such as actos® (pioglitazone, Takeda Pharmaceuticals North America, Inc.) that work at different receptors in the body. This is why regular monitoring of fasting insulin levels can be useful in detecting how the individual is responding to the medication.

Several studies have examined energy restricted diets without metformin and its effects on improving PCOS and weight loss (11,24,36-37). In all of the studies where weight loss was achieved, almost all lab parameters were improved. It does appear that weight loss can lower levels of insulin, testosterone, LH, and improve SHBG and menstrual function; women don't need to lose a lot of weight in order to see improvements. In fact, many studies suggest that even a moderate weight loss of 5% of total body weight can improve metabolic abnormalities of PCOS including insulin sensitivity and reproductive function (11,37). Similarly, it has been suggested that a 4% weight loss of total body weight can be beneficial in improving glucose regulation among individuals who are diabetic (57). This means that a woman with PCOS who weighs 220 pounds can expect to see improvements in her labs and symptoms, plus experience more regular menstrual cycles if she loses 11 pounds.

WEIGHT LOSS TO IMPROVE PCOS: IS IT NECESSARY?

It has been proven that weight loss is beneficial in improving virtually all clinical and reproductive parameters in women with PCOS. However, weight loss among the PCOS population is very difficult to achieve and requires the need for effective lifestyle interventions that do not require weight loss. This is particularly important as 70% of women with PCOS are obese (26). Dieting is known to have a high failure rate, plus most diets are not maintained for long periods of time. The majority of the people who do lose weight tend to regain it. Weight cycling has been known to worsen health and contribute to diet failure (11). Likewise, dieting leads to binge eating, poor body image and self-esteem and creates negative attitudes toward food and weight, all of which can affect an individual's future ability to make healthy dietary and lifestyle changes.

Studies show that some lab parameters worsen in PCOS individuals who regularly engage in binge eating, and improve when normalized eating is resumed (58). Both health professionals and patients need to ask themselves if it is worth it for a woman with PCOS, who has struggled with her weight her whole life, to risk worsening her condition and cause further medical complications by dieting. Are there effective interventions that do not require weight loss that can improve PCOS?

The answer: it depends on the individual and their goals. From clinical experience, I have worked with numerous women with PCOS who have been able to improve some of their lab parameters such as insulin, TG, cholesterol, LDL, and testosterone without losing any weight. It is possible and some studies have documented this (36,59). Patients have been able to improve these labs by engaging in regular physical activity and making changes to their diet, many of whom were also taking metformin.

One study looked at the role of diet in treating PCOS without a calorie restriction to see if changes in diet can improve PCOS independent of weight loss (36). In this study, 11 participants followed either a standard diet consisting of 56% of carbohydrates, 16% protein, and 31% fat, a MUFA diet consisting of 55% carbohydrates, 15% protein, and 33% fat, or a low carbohydrate diet of 43% carbohydrate, 15% protein, and 45% fat. All of the diets were approximately

2,000 calories and met the American Heart Association guidelines for cholesterol (under 300 mg) and fiber (25-30 grams per day) and were followed for 16 days each. Fasting insulin and TG were lower following the reduced carbohydrate diet (36). However, no change in fasting glucose or reproductive hormones was found. These results suggest that a eucaloric diet consisting of moderate CHO intake (approximately 43% total calories) combined with 45% fat (18% MUFA, < 8% saturated) with low cholesterol and high fiber can improve fasting insulin and TG of some women with PCOS without weight loss (36). Yet, for women who want to achieve pregnancy, it does appear that some weight loss may be needed to improve reproductive function (12,34,37).

EXERCISE AND PCOS

Physical activity has long been accepted as a key part in weight management and lifestyle modification and overall maintenance of physical and emotional health. PCOS women can certainly benefit from regular exercise since it can improve lipid levels, reduce insulin levels and improve insulin sensitivity and HTN. In addition, it can aid in the prevention and treatment of chronic diseases. It may also improve self-esteem, depression, and anxiety.

Included as part of its dietary guidelines, the USDA advises Americans to engage in 60 minutes of daily moderate-vigorous physical activity to maintain weight and prevent weight gain and 60 to 90 minutes of moderate-vigorous activity to lose weight and sustain weight loss. It has been shown that intermittent exercise (10-15 minute increments) throughout the day can be just as effective as continuous exercise with regards to weight management and may facilitate greater compliance to PCOS individuals who perceive continuous physical activity as a barrier (11).

Both aerobic and strength (resistance) training are effective methods for weight management and improving insulin sensitivity; they are important components to the treatment of PCOS (11). While aerobic exercise is beneficial in energy expenditure, strength training can be equally beneficial as it can increase resting metabolic rate and preserve or increase lean body mass. Strength training may be seen as a preferred choice of physical activity, especially among those with negative views toward traditional exercise. Additionally, strength training when combined with aerobic exercise, results in a greater improvement of insulin sensitivity than with aerobic exercise alone (60,61). Improvements may result from reductions of abdominal fat and maintenance of lean body mass (60). It is well known that androgens and anabolic steroids have been used to increase muscle size and strength. A positive relationship has been demonstrated between serum androgen levels and upper body-fat distribution in PCOS; muscle size in the leg is enhanced more than in the trunk region (62).

It seems as if regular exercise can even improve insulin sensitivity in PCOS, without losing weight. In a 3-month exercise program, 19 sedentary women with PCOS and insulin resistance showed a 25% improvement of insulin sensitivity without weight loss (59). The monitored exercise program was of moderate intensity, equivalent to walking briskly for an hour, 4 days per week.

Evidence clearly demonstrates the importance of physical activity for any PCOS woman, regardless of her weight status. Clients need to be educated on the benefits of regular physical activity for health and weight management. Dietitians should support clients to engage in aerobic and strength training exercises that are acceptable and physically comfortable for them to do. Ideally, activities should be viewed as fun and enjoyable for long-term compliance. Participation in daily lifestyle activities such as climbing stairs instead of taking the elevator, parking one's car further away and walking down the hall instead of e-mailing should also be encouraged. Finally, the use of motivational interviewing can be an effective behavior modification technique used to overcome perceived barriers to exercise and can be used to set realistic goals and reinforce exercise patterns.

In summary, the primary treatment for PCOS is a combination of lifestyle modification through diet and exercise. The use of insulin-sensitizers may be used in conjunction with lifestyle modification, not as a substitute. MNT plays an integral role in preventing and treating the clinical manifestations associated with PCOS. Therefore, dietetic professionals need adequate knowledge and training in working with the PCOS population. To date, low carbohydrate diets have not been proven to be superior to other diets in improving PCOS. The optimal diet for PCOS is one that reduces hyperinsulinemia and dyslipidemia, plus decreases the risk for chronic disease (15). A lower carbohydrate diet with an emphasis on whole grains, lean proteins, and omega-3 fatty acids is the best dietary composition to achieve this. Examples of eating plans for PCOS can be found in the appendix.

CHAPTER SUMMARY

- Weight loss is beneficial in improving all clinical parameters of PCOS and can improve reproductive function.
- High carbohydrate diets have been shown to worsen insulin resistance and triglycerides, and contribute to MBS.
- Low carbohydrate diets (<30%) have not been proven to be superior to other diets in improving PCOS.
- A moderately low GI diet can be beneficial in improving PCOS.
- Weight loss does not necessarily have to occur to improve insulin and lipid levels, however, it may be necessary to improve reproductive function.
- Regular screening of glucose tolerance, lipid levels, and blood pressure should be mandatory for all women with PCOS.
- Both aerobic and resistance training have been shown to improve insulin sensitivity independent of weight loss in PCOS women.

REFERENCES

1. Stein K. Polycystic Ovarian Syndrome: What It Is and Why Registered Dietitians Need to Know. *J Amer Diet Assoc.* 2006;106(11):1738-1741.
2. Scalzo K, McKittrick M. Response. *J Amer Diet Assoc.* 2000;100(8):957-958.
3. Case Problem: Dietary Recommendations to Combat Obesity,

Insulin Resistance, and Other Concerns Related to Polycystic Ovary Syndrome. *J Amer Diet Assoc.* 2000;100(8): 955-957.

4. Ehrmann DA, Liljenquist DR, Kasza K, Azziz R, Legro RS, Ghazzi MN. Prevalence and predictors of the metabolic syndrome in women with polycystic ovary syndrome. *J Clin Endocrinol Metab.* 2006;91:48-53.

5. Legro RS, Kunselman AR, Dodson WC. Prevalence and predictors of risk for type 2 diabetes mellitus and impaired glucose tolerance in polycystic ovary syndrome: a prospective, controlled study in 254 affected women. *J Clin Endo.* 1999;84:165-169.

6. Schroder A, Tauchert S, Ortmann O, Diedrich K, Weiss J. Insulin resistance in patients with polycystic ovary syndrome. *Ann Med.* 2004;3439.

7. Lord J, Thomas R, Fox B, Acharya U, Wilkin T. The effect of metformin on fat distribution and the metabolic syndrome in women with polycystic ovary syndrome–a randomised, double-blind, placebo-controlled trial. *Bjog.* 2006;113:817-24.

8. Pasquali R, Gambineri A, Biscotti D, Vicennati V, Gagliardi L, Colitta D, Fiorini S. Effect of long-term treatment with metformin added to hypocaloric diet on body composition, fat distribution, and androgen levels in abdominally obese women with and without the polycystic ovary syndrome. *J Clin Endo Metab.* 2000;85(8): 2767-2774.

9. Sharma S, Nestler J. Prevention of diabetes and cardiovascular disease in women with PCOS: treatment with insulin sensitizers. *Best Practice Research Clin Endo Metab.* 2006;20(2):245-260.

10. Feldeisen S, Tucker k. Nutritional strategies in the prevention and treatment of metabolic syndrome. *Appl Physiol Nut Metab.* 2007;32:46-60.

11. Moran LJ, Brinkworth G, Noakes M, Norman RJ. Effects of lifestyle modification in polycystic ovarian syndrome. *Reprod Biomed Online.* 2006;12:569-78.

12. Moran L, Norman RJ. Understanding and managing disturbances in insulin metabolism and body weight in women with polycystic ovary syndrome. *Best Practice Research Clin Endo Metab* 2004. 18(5):719-736.

13. Norman R, Davies M, Lord j. Moran L. The role of lifestyle modification in polycystic ovary syndrome. *Trends in Endo Metab.* 2002;13(6):251-257.

14. Pasquali R. Role of changes in dietary habits in polycystic ovary syndrome. *Reprod BioMed Online.* 2004;8(4):431-439.

15. Marsh K, Brand-Miller J. The optimal diet for women with polycystic ovary syndrome? *Br J Nutr.* 2005;94:154-65.

16. Orchard TJ TM, Goldberg R et al. The Effect of metformin and intensive lifestyle intervention on the metabolic syndrome: the Diabetes Prevention Program randomized trial. *Annals of Internal Medicine.* 2005;142:611-619.

17. Bruner B, Chad K, Chizen D. Effects of exercise and nutritional counseling in women with polycystic ovary syndrome. *Appl Physiol Nutr Metab.* 2006;31:384-91.

18. American association of clinical endocrinologists position statement on metabolic and cardiovascular consequences of polycystic ovary syndrome. *Endocrine Practice.*2005;11(2):125-134.

19. Apridonidze T, Essah PA, Iuorno MJ, Nestler JE. Prevalence and characteristics of the metabolic syndrome in women with polycystic ovary syndrome. *J Clin Endocrinol Metab.* 2005;90:1929-35.

20. Glueck CJ PR, Wang P, Goldenberg N, Sieve-Smith L. Incidence and Treatment of Metabolic Syndrome in Newly Referred Women with Confirmed Polycystic Ovarian Syndrome. *Metabolism.* 2003;52:908 -915.

21. US Department of Health and Human Services (DHHS), National Center for Health Statistics. *Third National Health and Nutrition Examination Survey (NHANES III), 1988-1994.* Hyattsville, MD: Center for Disease Control and Prevention; 1996.

22. Harborne L, Sattar N, Norman JE, Fleming R. Metformin and weight loss in obese women with polycystic ovary syndrome: comparison of doses. *J Clin Endocrinol Metab.* 2005;90:4593-4598.

23. McMillan-Price J, Petocz P, Atkinson f, O'Neill K. Comparison of 4 diets of varying glycemic load on weight loss and cardiovascular risk reduction in overweight and obese young adults. *Arch Intern Med.* 2006;166:1466-1475.

24. Douglas CC, Norris LE, Oster RA, Darnell BE, Azziz R, Gower BA. Difference in dietary intake between women with polycystic ovary syndrome and healthy controls. *Fertil Steril.* 2006;86:411-7.

25. Hirschberg AL, Naessen S, Stridsberg M. Impaired cholecysto-kinin secretion and disturbed appetite regulation in women with

polycystic ovary syndrome. *Gynec Endocinol.* 2004;19:79-87.

26. Cervero A, Dominguez F, Horcajadas, Quinonero A. The role of leptin in reproduction. *Curr Opin Obstet Gynecol.* 2006;18:297-303.

27. English PJ, Ghatei MA, Malik IA. Food fails to suppress ghrelin levels in obese humans. *J Clin Endocrin.* 2002;87:2984.

28. Moran LJ, Noakes M, Vlifton PM. Ghrelin and measures of satiety are altered in polycystic ovary syndrome but not differently affected by diet composition. *J Clin Endo Metab.* 2004;893337-3344.

29. Baranowska B, Radzikowska M, Wasilewska-Dziubinska E, Kaplinski A. Neuropeptide Y, leptin, galanin and insulin in women with polycystic ovary syndrome. *Gynecol Endocrinol.* 1999;13:344-351.

30. Jahanfar S, Malelki H, Mosavi AR. Subclinical eating disorder, polycystic ovary syndrome-is there any connection between these two conditions through leptin-a twin study. *Med J Malaysia.* 2005;60(4):441-6).

31. Sir-Petermann T. Polycystic ovary syndrome, a pathway to type 2 diabetes. *Nutrition.* 2005;21:1160-3.

32. Holte, J, et al. Restored insulin sensitivity but persistently increased early insulin secreion after weight loss in obese women with polycystic ovary syndrome. *J Clin Endocrinol Metabol.* 1995;80:2586-2593.

33. Carmina E, Legro RS, Stamets K, Lowell J,Lobo RA. Differences in body weight between American and Italian women with polycystic ovary syndrome: influence of the diet. *Hum Reprod.* 2003;18:2289-93.

34. Moran LJ, Noakes M, Clifton M, Tomlisson L, Norman RJ. Dietary composition in restoring reproductive and metabolic physiology in overweight women with polycystic ovary syndrome. *J Clin Endocrinol Metabol.* 2003;88:812-819.

35. Stamets K. A randomized trial of the effects of two types of short-term hypocaloric diets on weight loss in women with polycystic ovary syndrome. *Fert Steril.* 2004;81(3):630-7.

36. Douglas CC, Gower BA, Darnell BE, Ovalle F, Oster RA, Azziz R. Role of diet in the treatment of polycystic ovary syndrome. *Fertil Steril.* 2006;85:679-88.

37. Tolino A, Gambardella V, Caccavale C, D'Ettore A, Giannotti F, D'Anto V, De Falco CL. Evaluation of ovarian functionality after a dietary treatment in obese women with polycystic ovary syndrome. *Eur J Obstet Gynecol Reprod Biol.* 2005;119:87-93.

38. Moran LJ, Noakes M, Clifton PM, Wittert GA, Williams G, Norman RJ. Short-term meal replacements followed by dietary macronutrient restriction enhance weight loss in polycystic ovary syndrome. *Am J Clin Nutr.* 2006;84:77-87.

39. Willet WC. Dietary fat plays a major role in obestiy: no. Obes Rev. 2002;3:59-68.

40. Sloth B, Astrup A. Low glycemic index diets and body weight. *Inter J Obesity.* 2006;30:S47-S51.

41. Carels RA, Darby LA, Douglass OM, Cacciapaglia HM, Rydin S. Education on the glycemic index of foods fails to improve treatment outcomes in a behavioral weight loss program. *Eat Behav.* 2005;6:145-50.

42. Pittas AG, Das SK, Hajduk Cl, Golden J, Saltzman E, Stark PC. A low-glycemic index secretion but not in overweight adults with low insulin secretion in the CALERIE Trial . *Diabetes Care.* 2005; 28:2939-2941.

43. Fogli-Cawley J, Dwyer J, Saltzman E, McCullough M. The 2005 Dietary guidelines for Americans and insulin resistance in the framinhgam offspring cohort. *Diabetes Care.* 2007;30:817-822.

44. Ebbeling C, Leidig MM, Feldman HA, Lovesky MM, Ludwig DS. Effects of a low–glycemic load vs low-fat diet in obese young adults. *JAMA.* 2007;297:2092-2102.

45. Salermon J, Manson JE, Stampfer MJ, Colditz GA, Wing AL, Willett WC. Dietary fiber, glycemic load, and risk of non-insulin dependent diabetes mellitus in women. *JAMA.* 1997;277:472-477.

46. Slavin J. Whole grains and human health. *Nutrition Research Reviews.* 2004;17:1-12.

47. Ludwig DS. The glycemic index: physiological mechanisms relating to obesity, diabetes, and cardiovascular disease. *JAMA.* 2002;287:2414-2423.

48. Van Dam RM, Grievink L, Ocke MC, Feskens EJM. Patterns of food consumption and risk factors for cardiovascular disease in the general Dutch population. *Amer J Clin Nutr.* 2003;77:1156-1163.

49. McKeown NM MJ, Liu S, Saltzman E, Wilson PW, Jacques PF. Carbohydrate nutrition, insulin resistance, and the prevalence of the metabolic syndrome in the Framingham Offspring Cohort. *Diabetes Care.* 2004;27:538-46.

50. Appel LJ, Moore TJ, Obarzanek E. The DASH collaborative research group: A clinical trial of the effects of dietary patterns in blood pressure. *N Engl J Med* 1997; 336:1117-1124.

51. Ard, JD, Grambow SC, Liu D, Slentz CA. Draus WE, Sverkey LP. The effect of the PREMIER interventions on insulin sensitivity. *Diabetes Care.* 2004;27:340-347.

52. Hu FB, Stampfer MJ, Manson JE, Rimm E, Colditz GA, Rosner BA, Hennekens CH, Willett WC. Dietary fat intake and the risk of coronary heart disease in women. *N Engl J Med.* 1997; 337:1491-9.

53. Bhathena S. Relationship between fatty acids and the endocrine system. *BioFactors.* 2000;13:35-39.

54. Parillo M, Rivellese AA, Ciardullo AV, Capaldo B, Giacco A. Genovese S. A high-monounsaturated-fat/low-carbohydrate diet improves peripheral insulin sensitivity in non-insulin dependent diabetic patients. *Metabolism* 1992;41(12):1373-1378.

55. Expert Panel on Detection, Evaluation, and Treatment of High Blood Cholesterol in Adults. Executive Summary of the Third Report of the National Cholesterol and Education Program (NCEP) Expert Panel on Detection, Evaluation, and Treatment of High Blood Cholesterol in Adults (Adult Treatment Panel III). JAMA. 2001;285:2486-2497.

56. Mavropoulos J, Yancy W, Hepburn J, Westman EC. The effects of a low-carbohydrate, ketogenic diet on the polycystic ovary syndrome: a pilot study. *Nutr Metab.* 2005;2:35-40.

57. Knowler WC B-CE, Fowler SE et al. Reduction in the incidence of type 2 diabetes with lifestyle intervention or metformin. *New England Journal of Medicine.* 2002;346:393-403.

58. Morgan J, McCluskey S, Brunton JN, Lacey JH. Polycystic ovarian morphology and bulimia nervosa: a 9-year follow-up study. *Fert and Sterility.* 2002;77:928-31.

59. Brown AJ, Aiken LB, Setji T. Effects of exercise without weight loss on insulin resistance in women with polycystic ovary syndrome:a randowmized controlled study. *In 3rd Annual Meeting of the Androgen Excess Society* San Diego, CA. June 2005:28.

60. Cuff DJ. Meneilly GS, Martin A. Effective exercise modality to reduce insulin resistance in women with type 2 diabetes. *Diabetes Care.* 2003;26:2977-2982.

61. Eriksson J, Tuominen J, Valle T. Aerobic endurance exercise or circuit-type resistance training for individuals with impaired glucose tolerance? *Hormone and Metabolic Research.* 1998;30:37-41.

62. Douchi T, Yamamoto S, Oki T, Maruta K, Kuwahata R. Serum androgen levels and muscle mass in women with polycystic ovary syndrome. *Obstet Gynecol.* 1999;94(3):337-339.

CHAPTER 4

PRACTICAL APPLICATIONS

MEDICAL NUTRITION THERAPY AND THE ROLE OF THE DIETITIAN IN THE TREATMENT OF POLYCYSTIC OVARY SYNDROME

IT IS ESTIMATED THAT 31 to 35% of women with PCOS have impaired glucose tolerance (IGT) as well as a 7.5 to 10% prevalence of type 2 diabetes mellitus (T2DM) (1,2). The primary goals of treatment in PCOS are to normalize serum androgens and restore reproductive function. This is best achieved by improving insulin resistance through diet and lifestyle modification plus medication. Weight loss and reduction of abdominal fat result in improvement to most clinical and reproductive parameters, yet weight loss is very difficult for PCOS women to achieve. Most women with PCOS tend to have dyslipidemia and hypertension, thus requiring dietary guidelines that address these conditions. Additionally, because women with PCOS are at a higher risk for T2DM, coronary heart disease (CHD), and metabolic syndrome (MBS), diet composition must be aimed at preventing the onset of these conditions as well.

Currently, PCOS may be diagnosed more often than in the past because it has recently been classified as an endocrine disorder, not just a reproductive disorder. In addition, many women are frustrated with their symptoms and lack of results. Because of their frustration and their diagnosis, most of them have turned to the internet for advice where much of the information is false or misleading. It is expected that dietitians will treat more patients with PCOS, yet little attention has been given to the syndrome in professional publications where dietitians are the main audience. Education about the proper dietary management for PCOS is needed. This chapter discusses the use of medical nutrition therapy (MNT) for the treatment of PCOS, including diet composition and nutritional supplements. Sample meal plans using these recommendations can be found in the appendix. The role of the dietitian in treating PCOS is also discussed.

THE OPTIMAL DIET COMPOSITION FOR PCOS

Diet and lifestyle modifications, alone or in conjunction with medication, are seen as the primary treatment approaches for PCOS (3-7). The Diabetes Prevention Program (DPP) demonstrated that lifestyle modification through diet and exercise significantly reduced the risk of T2DM more than the insulin-sensitizer metformin (glucophage®, Bristol-Myers Squibb Co) (8).Weight loss, regardless of diet composition, has been shown to result in improvements of nearly all reproductive and metabolic parameters of PCOS (4, 9-12). Weight loss, however, is very difficult for the majority of women with PCOS to achieve. This demonstrates the need for effective diet strategies for PCOS, regardless of weight loss.

Currently, no formal dietary guidelines for PCOS exist. Traditionally, a high protein and low-carbohydrate (<30% total calories) diet has been thought to aid in weight loss and improve metabolic and reproductive dysfunction in PCOS (4,10,13). However, as discussed in Chapter 3, this diet composition has not been proven to be superior to other diets in improving PCOS. In one study, 28 overweight or obese women with PCOS followed a high-protein or low-protein diet consisting of 1400 calories each (10). After 3 months, both groups showed similar results in improving insulin, testosterone, and other hormone levels regardless of diet composition. While menstrual function was improved in both groups, no significant difference in weight loss was found (10). These findings are supportive of other studies that used a similar study design to compare high versus low protein diets (9,11).

The use of low-fat diets may not be the ideal diet composition for PCOS as they can increase triglyceride levels, decrease HDL concentrations, and worsen blood pressure (3,13). Low-fat recommendations may in fact promote a higher consumption of refined carbohydrates, especially because manufacturers tend to add sugar to reduced fat products. Too little fat in the diet can contribute to hunger, overeating, and weight gain as fat contributes to satiety. In contrast, diets rich in monounsaturated fatty acids (MUFAs) and polyunsaturated fatty acids (PUFAs) can improve the health of women with PCOS. A large, prospective study found that substituting MUFAs and PUFAs for just 5% of saturated fat calories reduced the risk of coronary heart disease in women by 42%. It was also found that replacing saturated fats with unsaturated fats was more effective in preventing coronary heart disease than decreasing overall fat intake (14). Consumption of omega-3 fatty acids has been demonstrated to improve insulin resistance (15), MBS and T2DM and subsequently PCOS, since these fatty acids have the ability to reduce triglycerides and LDL concentrations, increase HDL concentrations, lower blood pressure and glucose levels, and improve insulin sensitivity (3,16).

It has been shown that individuals with elevated insulin levels respond favorably to diets that modify carbohydrate content (17,18). Ebbeling et al. measured the insulin levels of obese adults without diabetes. One group was instructed to reduce carbohydrate intake to a maximum of 40% of calories and to consume only low-glycemic index (GI) foods. A second group was able to eat a variety of carbohydrate-containing foods (~55%) but had to limit fat intake to 20% of calories. Both groups reduced their calories by about 400 calories/day. After following the diets for 18 months, subjects with the highest insulin spikes at the beginning of the study lost a significant amount of weight (13 lbs on average) following the low GI diet. Those that followed the low-fat diet lost just an average of 3 lbs. In addition, the low GI diet was associated with greater improvements in HDL, LDL, and triglyceride levels than the low-fat diet (18).

These results suggest that moderate amounts of carbohydrates, if in the low GI form, can actually be beneficial to the treatment of PCOS; it can improve insulin sensitivity, glucose tolerance, hyperlipidemia, and overall MBS. Low GI foods contain more fiber and take longer to chew, which tends to increase satiety, reduce hunger, and lower subsequent voluntary food intake. In contrast, high GI foods have been known to stimulate appetite leading to greater food intake (7). Therefore, carbohydrates do not need to be avoided in the PCOS diet, but the type and quantity do have to be modified for optimal results. A diet low in saturated fat, rich in MUFAs and PUFAs and high in fiber from whole grain foods can improve both short and long-term symptoms of PCOS, as well as decrease risk of chronic diseases associated with insulin resistance. See Chapter 3 for more information on the health benefits of a low GI diet and the effects of other diet compositions on insulin resistance, MBS, and dyslipidemia in PCOS.

CARBOHYDRATES AND PCOS

THE DEFINITION OF A "LOW-CARBOHYDRATE DIET"

The International Food Information Council (IFIC) Foundation 2007 Food and Health Survey shows that more than half of Americans (55%) say they are concerned about the amount of carbohydrates they consume (19). Furthermore, 52% are concerned about the types of carbohydrates they consume, which is significantly higher than the previous year. Presently, the FDA does not have definitions for the terms "low-carbohydrate food," "net-carbs," or "low-carbohydrate diet." The U.S. Dietary Guidelines emphasize a daily carbohydrate intake of 45-65% of total calories. A diet composed of 35-40% carbohydrates would then be considered "low carb" (or "lower carb" as I prefer to call it). However, the American public may not share this same viewpoint.

From personal observation, I have noticed that many women with PCOS believe that they have to eat a very low-carbohydrate diet in order to lose weight and will expect the dietitian to give a meal plan that contains limited amounts of carbohydrates. This is partly due to poor dietary advice available on the internet and from misinformed health care providers. Thus, some part of nutrition sessions are usually spent educating PCOS clients on what is considered low-carbohydrate, and that diets extremely limited in carbohydrates are not particularly beneficial for PCOS. Usually, after I explain to my clients why I don't recommend these diets and the health risks associated with them, clients are more willing to give up their one-sided idea and even feel a bit relieved to know they can eat carbohydrate-containing foods and still improve their health.

RECOMMENDED AMOUNTS OF CARBOHYDRATES FOR PCOS

Carbohydrates are found in fruits, vegetables (mostly starchy ones), legumes, nuts, seeds, milk, and whole grains; they should be included as part of the healthy diet for PCOS. It is not advisable, nor healthy, for PCOS women to avoid vegetables, fruits or milk in the diet just because they contain carbohydrates. Due to their high fiber intake, fruits and starchy vegetables do not cause rapid rises in insulin secretion like refined carbohydrates, plus they provide numerous benefits to the metabolic profile of PCOS women (3). The DASH diet trials showed positive results for blood pressure, BMI, fasting glucose, triglycerides, and HDL cholesterol (20). Components of the DASH diet include high fruit and vegetable intake, whole grains, nuts, and low amounts of saturated fats and sweets. Although milk and legumes contain carbohydrates, they also provide a significant amount of protein which also limits the rise of insulin secretion. Vitamins and minerals derived from carbohydrate-laden foods, such as magnesium, are important in regulating insulin secretion (21).

Despite the popularity of high-protein and low-carbohydrate diets, it has been established that regular consumption of whole grains is beneficial to human health. In fact, the 2005 U.S. Dietary Guidelines recommend the consumption of at least 3 servings of whole grains daily, which most American's fail to meet (22). Both the American Diabetes Association and The American Heart Association also endorse the benefits of whole grains. Consumption of whole grains has been known to prevent and improve hyperinsulinemia and MBS, as well as reduced risk of T2DM (22-24). This evidence supports the need for whole grains to be included in the dietary recommendations for the treatment of PCOS.

Currently, there are no formal dietary guidelines for carbohydrate amounts in PCOS. As discussed in Chapter 3, too many carbohydrates consumed, especially if in the refined form, are not beneficial to health. However, evidence does not support severely limiting carbohydrate intake either as a dietary strategy to improve PCOS (9-11). From clinical experience, I have observed many women with PCOS experiencing strong carbohydrate cravings as well as hypoglycemic episodes. Dieting and binge eating are common for these women. I find that consuming moderate amounts of carbohydrates help ameliorate these issues. Usually, I will recommend my clients with PCOS consume a lower carbohydrate intake of approximately 35 to 40% of total daily calories (Table 1 lists the ranges of carbohydrates in grams based on caloric level). This carbohydrate intake is lower than the U.S. Dietary Guidelines but not so low that it limits the benefits from carbohydrate-containing foods. These are suggested guidelines and do not apply to all women. When recommending dietary guidelines for women with PCOS, it is important that they are individualized after assessing diet intake, activity level, eating disorder behaviors, medical concerns, and readiness to change.

Table 1. Suggested carbohydrate amounts for PCOS depending on caloric intake	
Daily Caloric Intake	Daily Carbohydrate Ranges (grams/day)*
1400	123-140
1600	140-160
1800	158-180
2000	175-200
2200	193-220
2400	210-240
*Based on a carbohydrate intake of 35-40% total caloric intake.	

Almost all carbohydrate-laden grain products (for example, pasta, rice, crackers, bread) should be whole grains. I use the term "almost all' because it is impossible to be a perfect eater, however, it is important that refined foods be limited as much as possible. Once consumed, refined carbohydrates cause greater spikes in insulin secretion compared to whole grains. Over time, this can worsen insulin resistance in PCOS, promoting T2DM (23-25). Additionally, consumption of refined carbohydrates tends to lead toward a greater intake of food overall. It is certainly acceptable and realistic for patients to have refined carbohydrates periodically, especially at special occasions (think birthday cake) as long as refined carbohydrates are limited or avoided at all other times. Furthermore, advising patients not to eat any refined carbohydrates creates an all-or-nothing mentality that can set people up for binge eating. On the other hand, sweetened beverages (juice, regular soda, sports drinks, sweetened iced tea) should be limited or avoided, as they provide little or no nutritive benefits and cause rapid increases in insulin levels.

It is important for carbohydrate-containing foods to be spread out evenly throughout the day, for example, between 3 small meals and snacks instead of consuming large amounts of them at one time. This will help control insulin levels, prevent hypoglycemia, and add to satiety with meals. Waiting too long between meals can be detrimental as it can lead to hypoglycemia and greater food intake, typically from carbohydrate-containing foods which can worsen insulin levels. For this reason, I usually advise my patients to eat every 3 to 5 hours. Adding protein sources to carbohydrate-containing foods seems to also help stabilize blood sugar levels longer between meals.

THE WHOLE GRAIN TRUTH

A whole grain consists of three layers: the bran, the endosperm, and the germ. The germ, or embryo, is the innermost part that contains vitamins E and K, essential oils, minerals, and protein. The endosperm makes up the majority of the grain with its center starchy part, whereas the bran makes up the outer layer consisting of fiber, protein, B-vitamins, and minerals. Often the outer two layers, the bran and the endosperm, are removed to produce a refined product. This process not only gives the grain a finer texture but it increases its shelf life. However, in removing the outer two layers, dietary fiber, vitamins, minerals, and phytochemicals are lost. Many times manufacturers "enrich" refined grains, adding back B-vitamins (niacin, thiamin, folic acid, and riboflavin) and iron to equal or greater than the amounts lost. Phytochemicals, antioxidants and fiber that are present in the whole grain are not added back to the refined grain. If the grain does not go through the refining process and its three layers remain completely intact, it is considered a "whole grain".

TYPES OF GRAINS

Whole grains are unique types of food due to their nutrient composition that consists of fat, protein, carbohydrates, vitamins, and minerals. Whole grains have been used as a staple in the diet for centuries, dating back to 12,000 B.C. Wheat, corn, rice, oats, rye and barley are common whole grains consumed in the U.S. Other grains such as spelt, millet, kamut, and quinoa are rapidly rising in popularity among health-conscious consumers. In fact, most, if not all of these grains can be found on the shelves of any grocery store (Whole Foods™ has some grains located in large bins in the front of its store, making them hard to miss). Yet, most of these whole grains are new to consumers who are not sure how to cook them or incorporate them into their diets. Therefore, it is important for dietitians not only to encourage the intake of whole grains but also be familiar with the different types including taste and cooking methods. Below are some descriptions of whole grains including their nutrient profile and suggestions for their use. Menus that incorporate some of these grains can be found in the appendix.

Amaranth. A staple of the Incas and the Aztecs, amaranth is a tiny grain, yellowish-brown in color that packs a hefty nutritional profile. Its seeds have more protein, iron, potassium, phosphorous, calcium, and magnesium than any other grain. In addition, it naturally has more of the amino acids lysine, methionine, and cysteine, which tend to be limited in other grains. Amaranth has a nutty flavor that emerges especially when it is toasted before grinding. The seeds can be used in bread recipes or popped like popcorn and eaten as a snack. If ground into flour, amaranth can be used if mixed with other flours in baking. Nutrition profile (1/4 cup, dry): 170 calories, 29 grams carbohydrates, 3 grams fiber, 7 grams protein, 2 grams fat.

Bulgur. Also referred to as cracked wheat, bulgur is considered a pseudograin that begins as a whole wheat kernel but is boiled, dried and cracked into small pieces, removing 5% of the bran. It is a staple in Middle-Easterners' diets and is the main ingredient in tabouli. Bulgur has a nutty, chewy texture. It is easy to prepare as it does not need to be washed before cooking and does not require stirring. It can be cooked in the microwave or stovetop. Bulgur swells during cooking requiring an adequate sized pot. It can be used in meatloafs, soups, stews, casseroles, and baked goods. Nutrition profile (1/2 cup, cooked): 76 calories, 17 grams carbohydrates, 4 grams fiber, 0 grams fat, 3 grams protein.

Flaxseed. Cultivated as early as 3,000 B.C., flaxseed is now a household name and it provides numerous nutritional benefits. Flaxseeds provide protein, vitamins, minerals, soluble and insoluble fiber, phytoestrogens, and is an excellent source of essential fatty acids. One tablespoon of ground flaxseeds meets the daily nutrient requirement for ALA, providing 1.8 grams. Flaxseeds are best digested when ground (use a coffee grinder) and should be stored in an airtight container in the refrigerator. Flaxseed can be used alone or as flour and are used in breads, muffins, crackers, and cereals. Milled flaxseed can be substituted for shortening or other oils and eggs (for every egg being replaced, mix 1 Tablespoon of milled flax with 3 tablespoons water). Nutrition profile (1 Tablespoon, ground): 36 calories, 2.7 grams carbohydrate, 2.2 grams fiber, 1.7 grams protein, 3.3 grams fat.

Kamut. "Kamut" is an ancient Egyptian word that means wheat. It has a buttery, nutty flavor and is a close relative to durum. It contains 8 amino acids, making it one of the grains with the highest protein content. It is also rich in vitamin E and B-vitamins. Kamut is mostly found in bread products such as cereals, crackers, and pasta. Nutrition profile (1/2 cup, cooked): 110 calories, 26 grams carbohydrates, 2 grams fiber, 3.5 grams protein, 1 gram fat.

Millet. There are over 6,000 varieties of millet. Its tiny, round and yellow kernels contain high amounts of protein, B-vitamins, vitamin E, calcium, iron, and phosphorous plus the oil present in it is 50% polyunsaturated. It contains more calories than wheat because of its higher oil content. Millet has a similar texture to wild rice and has a mild flavor that make it very versatile. It can be used as an ingredient in side dishes such as rice pilaf and stuffing, or used as porridge. Nutrition profile (1/4 cup, dry): 150 calories, 34 grams carbohydrates, 3 grams fiber, 5 grams protein, 2 grams fat.

Quinoa. Pronounced KEEN-wa, quinoa is the powerhouse of grains that has quickly risen in popularity among consumers due to its excellent nutrition profile, texture, and ease of use. Its seeds are small, flat and rounded and are similar to that of sesame seeds. Quinoa has a nutty taste with a soft, crunchy texture. It provides all essential amino acids, making it a complete protein food and has approximately twice as much protein as regular cereal grains. It is also rich in B-vitamins, vitamin A, magnesium, phosphorous, iron, fiber, calcium, and is relatively high in unsaturated fat (7%). Quinoa is technically not a grain but a fruit. It can be easily prepared and can be a great alternative to couscous or rice. Quinoa can be used to make pilafs, risottos, stews, salads, or even desserts. It can also serve as an excellent high-protein breakfast served hot, mixed with berries, nuts, or cinnamon. Its seeds must be rinsed first prior to cooking to remove its bitter saponin, a waxy protective coating. Nutrition profile (1/4 cup, dry): 140 calories, 25 grams carbohydrates, 4 grams fiber, 5 grams protein, 2 grams fat.

Spelt. Spelt is rich in B-vitamins and contains 8 essential amino acids. It has a sweet and nutty taste with a chewy texture. It is a slow-cooked grain that can be used in soups and stews like barley can and be easily be substituted in recipes calling for rice. Spelt can also be used as an ingredient in cookies, quick breads, and muffins. Nutrition profile (1/2 cup, cooked): 100 calories, 26 grams carbohydrates, 3.5 grams fiber, 4 grams protein, 1 gram fat.

SHOPPING FOR WHOLE GRAINS

Now that consumers are recognizing the benefits of whole grains and are becoming more "carb-selective" than ever before, manufacturers are trying to capitalize on the interest by using clever marketing strategies to lure consumers into bringing products into their homes. Some manufacturers even use coloring agents in their products to give them more whole grain attributes. Never before has it been more important to read the ingredient list on a product. Just because a label may say "100% wheat" or "multigrain" does not mean it is a whole grain product. The product is only considered whole grain if a whole grain such as bulgur, graham flour, oatmeal, whole-grain corn, whole oats, whole rye, whole wheat, or wild rice is listed as the first ingredient on the label's ingredient list. If a food is labeled, "stone-ground", "wheat flour", "seven-grain", or "bran" they are usually not a whole grain product.

The non-profit Whole Grains Council (www.wheatfoods.org) has developed a Whole Grain Stamp indicating if a food is mostly whole grain or not; it is now displayed on over 900 products. The stamp is distinctive with a black and gold print and is easy to identify on packages, making it a trustworthy symbol to consumers regardless of the brand. To qualify for the stamp, each food product must contain at least 51% of whole grains per serving.

WAYS TO ADD WHOLE GRAIN FOODS TO THE DIET

- Include a whole grain cereal, quinoa, or plain oatmeal with breakfast or snacks
- Add whole grains to dishes, such as barley in vegetable soup and stews or add prepared bulgur or flaxseed to waffles, pancakes, muffins, or baked goods for a nutty flavor
- Make sandwiches with whole grain bread
- Substitute pastas make with whole grain for regular pasta
- Try quick-cooking versions of brown rice, barley, and whole wheat couscous as side dishes to meals
- Use rolled oats or a crushed whole grain cereal to bread chicken, fish, or veal.
- Snack on whole grain crackers or "light" popcorn

DIETARY FIBER

It is recommended that women under the age of 50 consume approximately 25 grams of fiber daily. This can be easily met though the PCOS carbohydrate recommendations mentioned here that encourage regular consumption of fruits, vegetables, nuts, seeds, legumes, and whole grains. Dietary fiber aids in weight management by taking longer to chew thus giving a feeling of fullness while providing almost no calories. Additionally, a fiber-rich diet is important for proper digestion and can help lower the risk of heart disease and diabetes.

Both insoluble and soluble fibers are important to the health of PCOS women. Soluble fiber, found in foods such as oats, beans, apples, carrots, and barley, dissolves easily in water to form a gel and helps lower cholesterol and aids in blood sugar control. According to the National Heart, Lung, and Blood Institute's National Cholesterol Education Program (NCEP) Expert Panel, consuming 10 to 25 grams of soluble fiber will maximize LDL cholesterol reduction (26). In contrast, insoluble fiber (roughage) remains relatively intact, increasing movement throughout digestion by adding to stool bulk. Common food sources of insoluble fiber are whole wheat foods, wheat bran, nuts, and many vegetables.

The term "net-carbs" has become a popular phrase established in part by clever marketing of food companies to encourage consumption of their product. "Net carbs" is presumably established by subtracting fiber grams (or non-digestible carbs) from the total amount of carbohydrate per serving. Since the FDA does not currently define the term "net carbohydrates," I don't advise patients to use this method and find it only adds to more confusion in regards to food exchanges. Reading food labels and selecting foods high fiber with at least 3 grams per serving should, however be encouraged.

RECOMMENDED PROTEIN INTAKE FOR PCOS

A higher protein intake is needed to replace some carbohydrates in the diet. Protein takes longer to digest than carbohydrates thus adding to satiety (27) and requires less insulin to process, helping to keep insulin levels lower. In fact, clients should consume a protein source with all of their meals and snacks to help stabilize blood sugar levels and prevent hypoglycemia. Examples include a whole grain English muffin with egg, whole grain crackers and peanut butter, or cottage cheese and fruit. Because some protein foods tend to contain a significant amount of saturated and *trans* fat, it is best to encourage consumption of lean protein sources such as fish, turkey, skinless poultry, low-fat diary products, eggs, plus plant-based proteins such as soy, legumes, grains and vegetables. Generally, I will advise clients to consume approximately 15-30% of total calories from protein. However, it is best for clients to "experiment" with different amounts of protein in combination with other foods, to see what amount works best for them. This requires proficiency in mindful eating.

In addition to being low in saturated fat and free of cholesterol, soy has been shown to help reduce cholesterol levels. Government guidelines suggest that approximately 25 grams of soy protein be eaten daily to reduce cholesterol as part of a heart healthy diet. Soy foods like tofu, soy nuts, tempeh, edamame, soy milk and soy cheese are complete proteins and are also rich in B-vitamins and fiber as well as phytoestrogens, all of which are beneficial to PCOS women.

Phytoestrogens mimic estrogen in the body and possess antioxidant activity. The use of soy has been associated with improved ovarian function. In one study, anovulation improved in non-PCOS women who used black soybean powder in their diets (28). Soy is an excellent substitute for animal protein. Despite soy's rise in popularity, many people still are not sure how to cook with it or incorporate it into meals. Extra-firm tofu, for example, requires water to be pressed out in order to be successfully used in stir-fry's or grilled (it falls apart otherwise). A great website for recipes using soy products is www.soyfoods.com. The following are some suggestions to encourage clients add soy to their diets:

- Use extra-firm tofu in place of steak or chicken in stir-fry's
- Grilled (extra-firm) tofu or soy meatballs can be added to pasta dishes
- Soymilk can be used in cereals for breakfast or snacks
- Snack on soynuts or add it to trail mix
- Soy yogurt can be used in place of regular for breakfast and snacks
- Snack on steamed edamame or use it as a side dish or add it to salads
- Spread soy nut butter on whole-grain bread or apples instead of peanut butter
- Replace ricotta cheese with silken tofu in stuffed shells or lasagna
- Use soy-burgers in place of hamburgers

RECOMMENDED FAT INTAKE FOR PCOS

Because of a higher incidence of high triglycerides, elevated LDL and total cholesterol and low levels of HDL, women with PCOS would benefit from a diet rich in monounsaturated fats (olive oil, canola oil, peanuts, avocados, olives) and omega-3 fatty acids (fish, flaxseed, walnuts, soy). The consumption of saturated and *trans* fat should be limited. Currently, the NCEP recommends that no more than 7% of total daily calories come from saturated fat, up to 20% of daily calories from monounsaturated fatty acids, and up to 10% polyunsaturated fatty acids (26). However, like protein, total dietary fat needs may need to be increased for PCOS to compensate for the lower carbohydrate intake and to improve metabolic profile. For these reasons, I recommend clients' dietary fat intake be approximately 35-45% of total daily calories.

Research now shows that substituting unsaturated fats for saturated fats has more impact on reducing cholesterol and the risk of heart disease than does reducing the total amount of fat. Furthermore, consuming unsaturated fats has a greater effect on lowering cholesterol levels than does substituting carbohydrates for saturated fats. Omega-3 fatty acids in particular are known for their postprandial triglyceride-lowering effects, as well as reducing fasting levels. The Institute of Medicine recommends that Americans consume an ALA intake of 1.3 to 2.7 grams daily, on the basis of a 2000-calorie diet (29). The World Health Organization and North Atlantic Treaty Organization (WHO-NATO) recommend consuming 0.3 to 0.5 grams daily of eicosapentaenoic acid (EPA) and docosahexaenoic acid (DHA) (30). This can easily be met by consuming two servings of fatty fish twice a week (4 ounces each) and including plant sources of omega-3 fatty acids daily. One tablespoon of flaxseed meets the daily nutrient requirement for ALA, providing 1.8 grams. Women with a history of heart disease or high triglycerides should discuss the benefits of taking fish oil supplements with their doctors. A prescription is now available for a highly concentrated capsule form of omega-3's called Lovaza™ (Reliant Pharmaceuticals, Inc.). Lovaza™ is FDA-approved for treating hypertriglyceridemia (triglyceride levels of 500 mg/dL and above) in conjunction with dietary modifications. Lovaza™ contains 460 mg of EPA and 380 mg of DHA in 1 gram capsules.

Adding 2 grams daily of phytosterols (called plant sterols or stanols) to the diet has been shown to be effective in reducing LDL cholesterol levels by 13% (31). Phytosterols are now available in margarine spreads such as Take Control®, yogurts, as well as other foods and can be incorporated into a healthy eating plan.

Nutrition professionals need to help clients understand food labels. Now that the amount of *trans* fats are required to be on the Nutrition Facts panel for food products containing more than 0.5 grams of fat, it is easier for people to make healthier choices. However, just because a food claims to be *trans* free does not mean it is healthy. Indeed, many manufacturers eliminated *trans* fats from their products, yet as a substitute only added back palm kernel and other tropical oils. If palm kernel oil is listed among the first few ingredients, it will contain high amounts of saturated fat. Also, any food containing shortening, partially hydrogenated vegetable oil, intersterified, or stearate-rich oil contains *trans* fats and should be limited. Fast food, chips, crackers, baked goods, cereals, candy and energy bars are all common foods containing saturated and *trans* fats.

Although fat contains double the amount of calories per gram compared to carbohydrates or protein, it can be carefully added to a healthy eating plan. Dietitians should review portion sizes of fats and other foods with clients to prevent over consumption of fats and calories. Fat adds to satiety, keeping us satisfied longer and can prevent overeating. Many clients find they are less deprived when they have healthier fats at meals, which results in more long-term compliance. Dietary fats also provide a unique mouth feel and palatability to meals that carbohydrates and proteins do not. Ideally, each meal should include a source of fat, mostly unsaturated, to help meet suggested fat needs and to reduce the rise in insulin secretion following meals. The following are some easy ways for clients to meet the recommended dietary fat needs:

- Use canola or olive oil in cooking
- Add olives, nuts or seeds to salads
- Add avocado slices to sandwiches
- Snack on unsalted nuts
- Stir ground flax- seed into cereal, oatmeal, yogurt, or

smoothies
- Eat up to 12 ounces of fatty fish each week (salmon, mackerel, tuna)

RECOMMENDED SODIUM AMOUNTS FOR PCOS

Sodium intake should be consistent with government recommendations and limited to < 2,300 mg a day. Most Americans easily exceed this amount. Consuming too much sodium is associated with hypertension and can cause fluid retention. Diets that are highly refined and processed tend to be high in sodium. Results of the DASH diet trials indicated that elevated blood pressures were reduced by an eating plan that emphasizes fruits, vegetables, and low-fat dairy foods and is low in saturated fat, total fat, and cholesterol. The DASH eating plan includes whole grains, poultry, fish, and nuts with reduced amounts of fats, red meats, sweets, and sugared beverages. Whenever possible, clients should use no-added-salt, reduced-sodium or unsalted products (nuts, crackers) in place of regular ones. If applicable, fast food and dining out should be limited as well as the use of canned, boxed, and frozen foods. And, of course, avoid the salt shaker.

NUTRITIONAL SUPPLEMENTS FOR PCOS

While consuming a variety of foods should be sufficient to meet all required nutrient needs for most individuals, there are some nutrients that may be beneficial to PCOS women in higher amounts. The following are the most common and safest nutritional supplements I recommend to my PCOS clients. Clients should always discuss supplement use with their physicians prior to consumption. More information on these and other popular dietary supplements used among PCOS women, including recommended dosages can be found in Chapter 5.

CHROMIUM PICOLINATE

Although still not conclusive, supplementation of chromium picolinate may be effective in lowering glucose and insulin levels in people with T2DM, insulin resistance (32,33), and PCOS (34). A review of

15 studies on chromium supplementation showed that chromium deficiency results in insulin resistance (35). It was also concluded that insulin resistance due to chromium deficiency can be improved with chromium supplementation (35).

Research suggests that a combination of chromium picolinate and biotin is an effective adjunctive nutritional therapy for people with poorly controlled diabetes with the potential for improving lipid metabolism (36). A placebo-controlled, double-blinded, randomized trial examined the effect of chromium picolinate and biotin supplementation on glycemic control in 43 poorly controlled patients with type 2 diabetes mellitus (36). After 4 weeks, significant reductions in glucose and triglycerides were found compared to controls. Side effects of chromium picolinate are minimal, but it may cause hypoglycemia in patients taking diabetic medications.

CINNAMON CASSIA EXTRACT

This popular spice is believed to lower insulin, glucose, triglycerides and cholesterol levels in diabetics (37-40). One study demonstrated that intake of 1-6 grams of cinnamon daily for at least 40 days reduced serum glucose, triglyceride, LDL cholesterol, and total cholesterol levels in people with type 2 diabetes and therefore may also be beneficial in people with hyperinsulinemia (38). Cinnamon seems to work by increasing the phosphorylation of insulin receptors which leads to improved insulin function and improved insulin sensitivity (38). It may also reduce postprandial insulin response by delaying gastric emptying (40). Since it may lower glucose and insulin levels, careful monitoring of blood sugar levels is important to prevent hypoglycemia. Cinnamon can be sprinkled on cereal, peanut butter sandwiches, oatmeal, and on other foods but should be taken in a capsule form to meet therapeutic dosages of 3-6 grams daily. No reported side effects are known, making the consumption of this spice a relatively safe alternative option for PCOS women.

OMEGA-3 FATTY ACIDS

Known for their role in treating mood disorders and depression, omega-3 fatty acids such as ALA, EPA and DHA, may be used with

PCOS to reduce insulin and triglyceride levels and reduce the overall risk of cardiovascular disease (41,42). Omega-3 fatty acids can also aid in regulating hormone levels (15). Clients should be advised on ways to regularly incorporate foods rich in all forms of omega-3 fatty acids into their diet. This would include eating two servings (4 ounces each) weekly of fatty types of fish such as salmon or tuna or fish oil supplements, nuts, flax, olive and canola oils.

MAGNESIUM

Research shows that a higher intake of magnesium is associated with a 31% lower risk of developing MBS in young adults (43) and may be beneficial to women with PCOS. Insulin is involved in the shift of magnesium in cells, suggesting that blood magnesium levels play a role in maintaining blood insulin and glucose levels (44). Taking magnesium may decrease low-density lipoprotein (LDL) and total cholesterol levels as well as improve high-density lipoprotein (HDL) levels (45). Evidence also suggests magnesium plays a role in lowering diastolic blood pressure in individuals with mild to moderate hypertension (46).

Studies show that many Americans have an inadequate magnesium intake (47-52). A low dietary magnesium intake is theorized to be attributed to Americans' higher intake of processed and refined foods which are low in magnesium (47). Dietary sources of magnesium include legumes, whole grains, vegetables (especially broccoli, squash, and green leafy vegetables), seeds, and nuts (especially almonds). Other sources include dairy products, meats, chocolate, and coffee. Routine testing for magnesium levels is suggested in individuals with insulin resistance and metabolic syndrome (21). In addition, a thorough dietary assessment can help the clinician assess patients' magnesium intake by questioning them about dietary patterns, vitamin and mineral use and use of other supplements (21). If a deficiency is suspected, supplementation may be indicated as well as eating magnesium-rich food sources on a daily basis (21).

VITAMIN D

It has been speculated that the majority of individuals in the U.S. are deficient in vitamin D (53). Deficiency of vitamin D not only causes poor bone mineralization but also has been implicated in numerous chronic diseases including diabetes, heart disease, and cancer. Overweight and dark skinned people are at a higher risk for a vitamin D deficiency (54). One study reports improvement in reproductive function with the addition of vitamin D. The vitamin has been found to be involved in follicle egg maturation and development (54). Few foods contain vitamin D besides milk fortified with vitamin D, eggs, liver, cereals with vitamin D added, and fatty fish. Many researchers believe the current recommended amount for vitamin D is set too low. I usually recommend that my PCOS clients who are overweight or obese consider taking a vitamin D supplement of 1,000 IU daily and have their blood levels checked annually by their physicians.

PHYSICAL ACTIVITY RECOMMENDATIONS FOR PCOS

Physical activity may be as important as diet modification for women with PCOS. Evidence clearly demonstrates the importance of physical activity for PCOS including improved lipid levels, insulin sensitivity, HTN, self-esteem, depression, and anxiety. It can aid in the prevention and treatment of chronic diseases.

The USDA advises Americans to engage in 60 minutes of daily moderate-vigorous physical activity to maintain weight and prevent weight gain and 60 to 90 minutes of moderate-vigorous activity to lose weight and sustain weight loss. For clients who do not engage in physical activity, I recommend beginning with any amount of time and activity that they can healthfully sustain. Intermittent exercise (10-15 minute increments) throughout the day can be just as effective as continuous exercise with regards to weight management, and may facilitate greater compliance to PCOS individuals who perceive continuous physical activity as a barrier (4). For clients who are already engaged in routine physical activity, it may be helpful for dietitians to encourage a variety of exercises or make activities more challenging, such as lifting heavier weights, adding intervals, or increasing speed or incline levels.

Both aerobic and strength (resistance) training are effective methods for weight management and improving insulin sensitivity. They both are important components to the treatment of PCOS (4). While aerobic exercise is beneficial in energy expenditure, strength training can be equally beneficial since it can increase resting metabolic rate and preserve or increase lean body mass. Strength training may be seen as a preferred choice of physical activity, especially among those with negative views toward traditional exercise. Additionally, strength training when combined with aerobic exercise, results in a greater improvement of insulin sensitivity than with aerobic exercise alone (55,56).

Just because a woman with PCOS is exercising regularly at 65-80% of maximum target heart rate, it does not necessarily indicate that she will lose weight. From clinical experience, I can tell you that I have worked with exercise physiologists, personal trainers, and even women who have trained for marathons (thin and obese) who lost minimal or no weight despite a vigorous exercise regimen. This does not mean they are unhealthy or that the exercise they are doing is ineffective. In fact, one study showed that regular exercise improves insulin sensitivity in women with PCOS, without any resulting weight loss (57). Dietitians may need to reassure clients that engaging in regular activity is just as important as diet modification for improving health. Reviewing lab results with clients can be helpful to maintain compliance and add encouragement in these cases.

Clients need to be educated about the benefits of regular physical activity for PCOS including weight management and overall maintenance of physical and emotional health. Dietitians need to encourage clients to engage in regular aerobic and strength training exercises that are acceptable and physically comfortable for them to do. Ideally, activities should be viewed as fun and enjoyable for long-term compliance. Participation in daily lifestyle activities such as climbing stairs instead of taking the elevator, parking one's car further away and walking down the hall instead of e-mailing should also be encouraged. Dietitians may find some clients are motivated to walk more if they use pedometers with the goal of reaching 10,000 steps daily. Finally, the use of motivational interviewing can be an effective behavior modification technique used to overcome perceived barriers to exercise and can be used to set realistic goals and reinforce exercise patterns.

THE ROLE OF THE DIETITIAN IN TREATING PCOS

Dietitians, because of their unique role in developing an ongoing relationship with their clients, may have an advantage with identifying women they suspect of having PCOS and recommending further diagnostic testing. A few simple questions added to the nutrition assessment for all non-menopausal women can help screen clients for PCOS. These questions include asking about weight history, menstrual cycle (absent, irregular, clots or heavy), if they experience any acne, hair loss, growth of hair on their faces, abdomen, inner thighs, or back. Table 2 lists some specific questions that can be used to screen patients for PCOS. If one or more of the answers are yes, dietitians may want to probe further, asking clients if they ever experience signs of low blood sugar, or food cravings, plus ask about a family history of PCOS, before recommending clients get proper testing done by their physicians.

Table 2. Questions Used to Screen Patients for PCOS:

"Tell me what your periods are like. Are they heavy, irregular, absent, etc.?"
"Do you ever feel lightheaded, dizzy, nauseous or irritability that gets better when you eat?"
"Have you ever been told by your physician or healthcare provider that you have any abnormal lab values?"
"Can you tell me about any excessive body hair that you've dealt with?"
"What types of foods do you crave and when do you crave them?"
"Do you have dry/rough elbows or any dark patches that look dirty on your body?"
"Does anyone in your family have polycystic ovary syndrome?"

In addition to exploring clients' eating habits and attitudes toward food and weight, dietitians should review laboratory tests with clients, ideally during the nutrition assessment. Laboratory tests should include lipid profile, fasting blood glucose, glycohemoglobin A1C (HA1C), and fasting insulin and androgen levels (see Chapter 1 for information on these and other labs used to diagnose and treat PCOS). I find that clients are very interested in knowing their metabolic profile and it can be a great motivational tool for clients to monitor improvements through laboratory results as they make changes to their eating and activity levels. It can also help clients relate to their symptoms better if they know what is going on inside their bodies.

Dietitians will also need to discuss medication and supplement use with their clients. The most common medications among PCOS women are birth control pills, antiandrogens such as spironolactone, and insulin-sensitizing agents such as metformin. Clients will need to be educated on the side effects of these medications, especially metformin, which may cause diarrhea and gastrointestinal upset in the first several weeks of starting it. It is also important for clients to understand that metformin is not a weight loss drug and is only effective if accompanied by diet and lifestyle modifications. Additionally, many women with PCOS seek out alternative treatments to conventional medicine involving herbal supplements. This can be problematic as herbal supplements can interact with medications and are not fully regulated by the FDA. For more information on common herbal and dietary supplements used by women with PCOS see Chapter 5.

Not only do clients need dietitians to educate them on healthful, balanced diets but they also need to be educated on the pathophysiology of PCOS, simplified as much as possible. Clients need to understand how the hormonal imbalance of PCOS is affecting their symptoms as well as the increased risks of heart disease and diabetes. Education should include the role of insulin in the body, what insulin resistance is, how insulin affects weight, that exercise benefits it, and how both the type and quantity of food affects insulin levels. Clients need to understand that the treatment of PCOS is aimed at lowering insulin levels and that the three most effective methods to do this are diet, exercise, and medications.

Dietitians should take an empathetic approach in counseling their PCOS clients (58). Many women are embarrassed and frustrated about their symptoms. It could be helpful to let clients know they are not alone in their diagnosis and that the symptoms they experience, including their struggles with weight, are very common among the PCOS population and are not their fault. It is also common for these women to feel hopeless; they need to know that changes in diet and lifestyle can make a difference even if not accompanied by weight loss. Dietitians can refer clients to therapists with experience in PCOS for mental health treatment and if available, PCOS support groups.

Generally, I find that women with PCOS tend to be motivated in wanting to make changes in their eating and improve their symptoms. Ultimately, clients' knowledge and understanding of their diagnosis should dictate the direction of nutrition sessions (58) including nutrition education and goal setting. Some clients are able to handle a lot of information at once and are able to implement changes after one session, whereas some clients may only be able to handle small bits of information at a time, setting just a few goals at each session.

THE DIETITIAN'S TOOLBOX

The following are some helpful tools dietitians may want to use in providing medical nutrition therapy with their PCOS clients:

Food models. The use of food models is a very effective way to educate clients on serving sizes of food. By actually viewing the portion size of a food, clients can better plan their meals and follow a meal plan (if they're on one). It is also very helpful for someone who eats out often to see what constitutes a serving.

Food records. Although many clients dislike them (probably associated from negative past experiences with dieting), food records are a very powerful tool for both clients and nutrition professionals. Keeping a daily account of food eaten can give the dietitian a better idea of what clients are eating and can be used to monitor their progress. It also helps clients become more aware and accountable of their own eating habits. Mostly though, I find that clients benefit from trying to connect to their levels of hunger and satisfaction before and after meals. It can be useful to challenge clients who describe their mood and feelings associated with eating, as it can help overcome distorted eating by the use of reality checks and uncovering connections between food and feelings.

The scale. Some clients may wish to monitor their weight regularly (once a week or every other week) to see if insulin levels have worsened or to reflect changes in eating. However, I usually discourage my PCOS clients from frequent weighing and will rarely weigh clients myself. This is especially true if their weight has been stable, they are active, not bingeing nor using any other eating disordered behaviors, and they are working at listening to internal appetite regulation. Weight loss can be very slow for most women with PCOS. Besides, most women can tell by their clothes if they are losing or gaining weight. Furthermore, I have seen many women with PCOS who improve their health without weight loss. Therefore, emphasis should be on improving metabolic fitness rather than weight loss.

In summary, dietitians play a crucial role in the recognition and treatment of PCOS. Lifestyle modification of diet and exercise are the primary treatment approaches for improving PCOS and preventing further health complications. A diet lower in whole grain carbohydrates, with lean protein sources and rich in MUFAs and PUFAs is the best way to achieve this. Treatment must be individualized according to clients' symptoms, health concerns, knowledge, and readiness to change. In addition to providing nutrition education on proper dietary recommendations, dietitians need to help clients understand the pathophysiology of PCOS and the health risks associated with the syndrome. Overall, clients need to be supported by dietitians to improve their health, with a focus on metabolic fitness rather than weight loss.

SUMMARY OF RECOMMENDED DIETARY GUIDELINES FOR THE TREATMENT OF PCOS:

- Consume a variety of foods
- Carbohydrate intake should be reduced to approximately 35-40% of total daily calories
- Almost all grain products should come from whole grains
- Avoid sweetened beverages
- Eat every 3 to 5 hours
- Protein intake should be approximately 15-30% of total

    daily calories
- Consume lean protein sources with all meals or snacks
- Daily fat intake should be approximately 35-45% of total daily calories. This includes no more than 7% of total daily calories coming from saturated fat. Trans fats should be eliminated
- Up to 20% of daily calories from monounsaturated fatty acids, and up to 10% polyunsaturated fatty acids
- Consume fatty fish (up to 12 oz./week) twice a week
- Consume a minimum of 25 grams of fiber each day
- Limit sodium intake to $\leq 2,300$ mg/day
- Vitamin D supplementation of 1,000 IU daily
- Consume soy products on a regular basis (ideally, 25 grams/day)
- Engage in daily physical activity

Menu plans that incorporate these guidelines can be found in the appendix.

REFERENCES

1. Ehrmann DA, Liljenquist DR, Kasza K, Azziz R, Legro RS, Ghazzi MN. Prevalence and predictors of the metabolic syndrome in women with polycystic ovary syndrome. *J Clin Endocrinol Metab.* 2006;91:48-53.

2. Legro RS, Kunselman AR, Dodson WC. Prevalence and predictors of risk for type 2 diabetes mellitus and impaired glucose tolerance in polycystic ovary syndrome: a prospective, controlled study in 254 affected women. *J Clin Endo.* 1999;84:165-169.

3. Feldeisen S, Tucker k. Nutritional strategies in the prevention and treatment of metabolic syndrome. *Appl Physiol Nut Metab.* 2007;32:46-60.

4. Moran LJ, Brinkworth G, Noakes M, Norman RJ. Effects of lifestyle modification in polycystic ovarian syndrome. *Reprod Biomed Online.* 2006;12:569-78.

5. Norman R, Davies M, Lord j. Moran L. The role of lifestyle modification in polycystic ovary syndrome. *Trends in Endo Metab.*

2002;13(6):251-257.

6. Pasquali R. Role of changes in dietary habits in polycystic ovary syndrome. *Reprod BioMed Online.* 2004;8(4):431-439.

7. Marsh K, Brand-Miller J. The optimal diet for women with polycystic ovary syndrome? *Br J Nutr.* 2005;94:154-65.

8. Orchard TJ TM, Goldberg R et al. The Effect of metformin and intensive lifestyle intervention on the metabolic syndrome: the Diabetes Prevention Program randomized trial. *Annals of Internal Medicine.* 2005;142:611-619.

9. Stamets K. A randomized trial of the effects of two types of short-term hypocaloric diets on weight loss in women with polycystic ovary syndrome. *Fert Steril.* 2004;81(3):630-7.

10. Moran LJ, Noakes M, Clifton M, Tomlisson L, Norman RJ. Dietary composition in restoring reproductive and metabolic physiology in overweight women with polycystic ovary syndrome. *J Clin Endocrinol Metabol.* 2003;88:812-819.

11. Douglas CC, Gower BA, Darnell BE, Ovalle F, Oster RA, Azziz R. Role of diet in the treatment of polycystic ovary syndrome. *Fertil Steril.* 2006;85:679-88.

12. Moran LJ, Noakes M, Clifton PM, Wittert GA, Williams G, Norman RJ. Short-term meal replacements followed by dietary macronutrient restriction enhance weight loss in polycystic ovary syndrome. *Am J Clin Nutr.* 2006;84:77-87.

13. Moran L, Norman RJ. Understanding and managing disturbances in insulin metabolism and body weight in women with polycystic ovary syndrome. *Best Practice Research Clin Endo Metab* 2004. 18(5):719-736.

14. Hu FB, Stampfer MJ, Manson JE, Rimm E, Colditz GA, Rosner BA, Hennekens CH, Willett WC. Dietary fat intake and the risk of coronary heart disease in women. *N Engl J Med.* 1997; 337:1491-9.

15. Bhathena S. Relationship between fatty acids and the endocrine system. *BioFactors.* 2000;13:35-39.

16. Parillo M, Rivellese AA, Ciardullo AV, Capaldo B, Giacco A. Genovese S. A high-monounsaturated-fat/low-carbohydrate diet improves peripheral insulin sensitivity in non-insulin dependent diabetic patients. *Metabolism* 1992;41(12):1373-1378.

17. Pittas AG, Das SK, Hajduk Cl, Golden J, Saltzman E, Stark PC. A low-glycemic index secretion but not in overweight adults with low

insulin secretion in the CALERIE Trial . *Diabetes Care.* 2005; 28:2939-2941.

18. Ebbeling C, Leidig MM, Feldman HA, Lovesky MM, Ludwig DS. Effects of a low–glycemic load vs low-fat diet in obese young adults. *JAMA.* 2007;297:2092-2102.

19. The International Food Information Council (IFIC) Foundation 2007 Food and Health Survey: Consumer attitudes toward food, nutrition, and health. Available at www.ific.org. Accessed on August 1, 2007.

20. Appel LJ, Moore TJ, Obarzanek E. The DASH collaborative research group: A clinical trial of the effects of dietary patterns in blood pressure. *N Engl J Med* 1997; 336:1117-1124.

21. Monahan Couch L. The role of magnesium-rich foods and magnesium supplementation in diabetes management. Pending publication in *Topics of Clin Nutr.* 2007.

22. Slavin J. Whole grains and human health. *Nutrition Research Reviews.* 2004;17:1-12.

23. Ludwig DS. The glycemic index: physiological mechanisms relating to obesity, diabetes, and cardiovascular disease. *JAMA.* 2002;287:2414-2423.

24. McKeown NM MJ, Liu S, Saltzman E, Wilson PW, Jacques PF. Carbohydrate nutrition, insulin resistance, and the prevalence of the metabolic syndrome in the Framingham Offspring Cohort. *Diabetes Care.* 2004;27:538-46.

25. Van Dam RM, Grievink L, Ocke MC, Feskens EJM. Patterns of food consumption and risk factors for cardiovascular disease in the general Dutch population. *Amer J Clin Nutr.* 2003;77:1156-1163.

26. Expert Panel on Detection, Evaluation, and Treatment of High Blood Cholesterol in Adults. Executive Summary of the Third Report of the National Cholesterol and Education Program (NCEP) Expert Panel on Detection, Evaluation, and Treatment of High Blood Cholesterol in Adults (Adult Treatment Panel III). JAMA. 2001;285:2486-2497.

27. Halton T, Hu F. The effects of high protein diets on thermogenesis, satiety and weight loss: a critical review. J Am College Nutr. 2004;23(5):373-385.

28. Kohama T, Kobayashi H, Inoue M. the effect of soybeans on the

anovulatory cycle. J med food. 2005;8(4):550-551.

29. Institute of Medicine's Dietary Reference Intake Database. Assessed June 29, 2007.

30. Kris-Etherton P, Harris WS, Appel LJ. Fish Consumption, Fish Oil, Omega-3 Fatty Acids, and Cardiovascular Disease. Am Heart Assoc Sci Statement. 2002; 2747-2757.

31. Cater NB, Garcia-Garcia AB, Vega GL, Grundy SM. Responsiveness of plasma lipids and lipoproteins to plant stanol esters. *Am J Cardiol.* 2005; 96:23D-28D.

32. Vladeva SV, Terzieva DD, Arabadjiiska DT. Effect of chromium on the insulin resistance in patients with type II diabetes mellitus. *Folia Med (Plovdiv).* 2005; 47:59-62.

33. A scientific review: the role of chromium in insulin resistance. *Diabetes Educ.* 2004; Suppl:2-14.

34. Lydic ML, McNurlan M, Komaroff E, et al. Effects of chromium supplementation on insulin sensitivity and reproductive function in polycystic ovarian syndrome: A pilot study. *Fertility and Sterility.* 2003;80:45-46(abstract).

35. Mertz W. Chromium in human nutrition: a review. *J Nutr.* 1993;123:626-63

36. Singer GM, Geohas J. The effect of chromium picolinate and biotin supplementation on glycemic control in poorly controlled patients with type 2 diabetes mellitus: a placebo-controlled, double-blinded, randomized trial. *Diabetes Technol Ther.* 2006; 8:636-43.

37. Anderson, R.A. 2005. Polyphenols from cinnamon increase insulin sensitivity: Functional and clinical aspects [abstract]. *Dietary Antioxidants, Trace Elements, Vitamins and Polyphenols.* 2005;4:154.

38. Khan A, Safdar M, Khan MMA, et al. Cinnamon improves glucose and lipids of people with type 2 diabetes. *Diabetes Care.* 2003;26:3215-3218.

39. Mang B, Wolters M, Schmitt B, Kelb K, Lichtinghagen R, Stichtenoth DO, Hahn A. Effects of a cinnamon extract on plasma glucose, HbA, and serum lipids in diabetes mellitus type 2. *Eur J Clin Invest.* 2006;36:340-4.

40. Hlebowicz J, Darwiche G, Bjorgell O, Olof L. Effect of cinnamon on postprandial blood glucose, gastric emptying, and satiety in healthy subjects. *Amer J Clin Nutr.* 2007;85(6):1552-1556.

41. Psota TL, Gebauer SK, Kris-Etherton P. Dietary Omega-3 Fatty Acid Intake and Cardiovascular Risk. The American Journal of Cardiology. 2006;98(4):3-18.

42. Riccardi G, Giacco R, Rivellese AA. Dietary fat, insulin sensitivity and the metabolic syndrome. *Clin Nutr.* 2004; 23:447-56.

43. He K, Liu K, Daviglus ML, Morris SJ, Loria CM. Magnesium intake and incidence of metabolic syndrome among young adults. *Circulation.* 2006;113:1675-1682.

44. Fung TT, Hu FB, Pereira MA, Liu S, Stampfer MJ, Colditz GA, Willett WC. Whole-grain intake and the risk of type 2 diabetes: a prospective study in men. *Am J Clin Nutr.* 2002;76:535-40.

45. Guerrero-Romero F, Rodriguez-Moran M. Hypomagnesemia is linked to low serum HDL-cholesterol irrespective of serum glucose values. *J Diabetes Complications.* 2000;14:272-6.

46. Jee SH, Miller ER, Guallar E, Sing VK, Appel LJ, Klag MJ. The effect of magnesium supplementation on blood pressure: a meta-analysis of randomized clinical trials. *Am J Hypertens.* 2002;14:691-696.

47. Lopez-Ridaura R, Willett WC, Rimm EB, Liu S, Stampfer MJ, Manson JE, Hu FB. Magnesium intake and risk of type 2 diabetes in men and women. *Diabetes Care.* 2004;27:134-40.

48. Ford ES, Mokdad AH. Dietary magnesium intake in a national sample of US adults. *J Nutr.* 2003;133:2879-82.

49. Dietary Guidelines for Americans 2005. Available at: http://www.health.gov/DietaryGuidelines/. Accessed on September 16, 2006.

50. Liese AD, Roach AK, Sparks KC, Marquart L, D'Agostino RB, Jr., Mayer-Davis EJ. Whole-grain intake and insulin sensitivity: the Insulin Resistance Atherosclerosis Study. *Am J Clin Nutr.* 2003;78:965-71.

51. Moshfegh A GJ, Cleveland L. What We Eat in America, NHANES 2001-2002; usual nutrient intakes from food compared to dietary reference intakes. 2005.

52. Kao W. Serum and Dietary Magnesium and the risk for Type 2 Diabetes Mellitus, The Atherosclerosis Risk in Communities Study. *Archives of Internal Medicine.* 1999;159:2151-2159.

53. Holick MF. Vitamin D: importance in the prevention of cancers, type 1 diabetes, heart disease, and osteoporosis. *Am J Clin Nutr.* 2004;79(3):362-71.

54. Thys-Jacobs S, Donovan D, Papadopoulos A, Sarrel P, Bilezikian JP. Vitamin D and calcium dysregulation in the polycystic ovarian syndrome. Steroids 1999;64(6):430-5.

55. Cuff DJ. Meneilly GS, Martin A. Effective exercise modality to reduce insulin resistance in women with type 2 diabetes. *Diabetes Care*. 2003;26:2977-2982.

56. Eriksson J, Tuominen J, Valle T. Aerobic endurance exercise or circuit-type resistance training for individuals with impaired glucose tolerance? *Hormone and Metabolic Research*. 1998;30:37-41.

57. Brown AJ, Aiken LB, Setji T. Effects of exercise without weight loss on insulin resistance in women with polycystic ovary syndrome:a randowmized controlled study. *In 3ʳᵈ Annual Meeting of the Androgen Excess Society* San Diego, CA. June 2005:28.

58. Case Problem: Dietary Recommendations to Combat Obesity, Insulin Resistance, and Other Concerns Related to Polycystic Ovary Syndrome. *J Amer Diet Assoc*. 2000;100(8): 955-957.

CHAPTER 5

ALTERNATIVE AND COMPLEMENTARY TREATMENTS

THE USE OF DIETARY AND HERBAL SUPPLEMENTS IN TREATING PCOS

TODAY, MORE AND MORE people in the United States are turning to alternative treatments and complementary medicine to improve their health. According to the National Institutes of Health (NIH) Office of Dietary Supplements, consumers spent $20.3 billion on dietary supplements in 2004. The trend is driven by several factors including increased availability of supplements, desire for control of one's own destiny, perception of increased safety, and disillusionment with traditional medicine. Many women with PCOS who have been misdiagnosed or have not seen improvement in their symptoms are frustrated with their medical care and it is not surprising, therefore, for them to turn to alternative treatments in hopes of getting better results.

As with all supplements there are numerous concerns, one of which is supplement-medication interactions. This is particularly important considering that most individuals do not reveal to their physicians that they are taking a dietary or herbal supplement. Many supplements and drugs utilize the same metabolic pathway in the liver, increasing the chances for an interaction which could alter the effect of the supplement or medication in the body resulting in serious side effects, even death. For instance, a greater vitamin K intake can oppose the action of the oral anticoagulant warfarin, leading to blood clots. Similarly, the popular antiandrogen medication, spironololactone (aldactone), is a potassium-sparing diuretic.

Taking potassium supplements in addition to spironolactone will cause blood levels of potassium to rise to dangerous levels, possibly resulting in heart failure and death.

Another major concern includes the safety of the supplements, considering there are not many well designed and controlled studies on them. The FDA does not monitor them nearly as closely as they do food or drugs. For example, ephedra, used in the past for weight loss and enhancement of athletic performance, was banned by the FDA in December, 2003 after it was found to cause fatal cardiac side effects such as tachycardia, arrhythmias, and hypertensive crisis (1).

As far as advertising laws are concerned, a dietary supplement cannot claim on its label that it will diagnose, cure, mitigate, treat, or prevent a disease. Manufacturers of a dietary supplement are allowed to have one of the following three claims on its label: a health claim (showing the relationship between an ingredient and ability to reduce risk of disease), nutrient content claim, structural or functional claim (how it may affect the body). These products must also have a disclaimer label that reads "This statement has not been evaluated by the FDA."

Currently, quality control of dietary supplements is a big safety concern as manufacturers do not have to provide the FDA with evidence of product safety. This means that dietary supplement manufacturing plants are not required to be inspected or monitored for quality control. Manufacturers may fabricate products with limited or no amounts of active ingredients (2). Consumers may be thinking they are getting the actual amount of the supplement that the label claims but in many instances, this may not be true. Additionally, cases have been reported in which products have been contaminated by pesticides, heavy metals, and other impurities. Rarely will a supplement be recalled unless the FDA has significant evidence of adverse risks.

However, starting in June 2008, all this will change thanks to a new ruling by the U.S. Food and Drug Administration. The current good manufacturing practices (CGMPs) final rule will require that proper controls be in place for dietary supplements so that they are processed in a consistent manner and meet quality standards (companies with less than 500 employees have until June 2009 and companies with fewer than 20 employees have until June 2010 to comply with the regulations) (2). The CGMPs apply to all domestic and foreign companies that manufacture, package, label or hold dietary supplements, including those involved with the activities of testing, quality control, packaging and labeling, and distributing them in the U.S. The rule establishes requirements that dietary supplements be manufactured consistently as to identity, purity, strength, and composition (2) allowing consumers to be confident that the products they purchase contain what is on the label. Additionally, all manufacturers will be required to report all serious dietary supplement adverse events to FDA by the end of 2007.

Many people may think that there is no harm to taking supplements as they may see them as "natural" or "safe" and this may cause them to exceed the dosage or combine them with other supplements or medications in hopes of improving the effectiveness of them. Therefore, it is important to properly screen PCOS clients for any supplement use and to inform clients of the risks of taking any dietary or herbal supplements. It is also imperative for them to inform their physicians of any supplements they may be taking.

Because a limited number of well-controlled scientific studies, such as randomized clinical trials, have been conducted on the effects of most herbal supplements, I am hesitant to recommend clients take them except for a small number of ones listed with minor side effects. Even then, careful monitoring of the supplement for any reaction is warranted. Also, I do not recommend any of these supplements to pregnant or lactating women or to women that may become pregnant, due to the risk of contamination of the product and potential adverse risks to the fetus. With that being said, I do think it is important that dietitians familiarize themselves with these supplements because they are rising in popularity among women with PCOS and because they could be beneficial in improving some PCOS symptoms. The following are some common dietary and herbal supplements used among women with PCOS as an alternative or adjunct to their current medical treatment.

Alpha-Lipoic Acid

Purported use: diabetes, insulin resistance
Recommended dosage: 600-1200 mg/day

Alpha-lipoic acid (ALA) is synthesized in mitochondria and is proposed to be an antioxidant. It is involved in carbohydrate metabolism and is believed to help lower blood glucose by its ability to help insulin move glucose into the body's cells. In fact, ALA has long been used in Germany to treat diabetic polyneuropathy (3,4). Yeast, liver, kidney, spinach, broccoli, and potatoes are good sources of alpha-lipoic acid. Doses of ALA up to 2,000 mg/day have reportedly been well tolerated, however, ALA should be used with caution as some side effects including skin reactions, GI upset, and possible hypoglycemia have been reported (4).

To date, no clinical studies have evaluated the use of ALA in PCOS. A placebo-controlled pilot trial involving supplementation of ALA among individuals with type 2 diabetes showed improvements in insulin sensitivity compared to controls. Seventy-four individuals were assigned a placebo or treatment of ALA in doses of 600 mg, 1,200 mg, or 1,800 mg (5). There was no dose response effect seen in the three different ALA treatment groups. The researchers suggest that oral administration of ALA can improve insulin sensitivity in patients with type 2 diabetes (5), and therefore, may be applicable to improving insulin sensitivity in PCOS.

Black Cohosh

Also known as Cimicifuga racemosa
Purported use: depression, lowering lutenizing hormone, regulating mood swings, normalizing irregular periods, menopause, PMS, reducing serum cholesterol
Recommended dosage: 40-80 mg standard extract 2x/day

Black cohosh is a plant found in Europe, North America and Asia whose roots and herbs act as phytoestrogens to mimic estrogen in the body. It is sold in capsules, tablets, tinctures, and teas. Remifemin, as it is commonly known, is available in the U.S. and is popular in relieving PMS and menopausal symptoms, especially hot flashes, and is an alternative to hormone replacement therapy (6). Although data are still conflicting, most clinical trials show that black cohosh is not effective in lowering lutenizing (LH) levels (7,8). The use of black cohosh is recommended to be limited to 6 months as long-term trials are lacking. Adverse reactions may include gastrointestinal upset, rash, headache, dizziness, weight gain, feeling of heaviness in the legs, cramping, and vaginal spotting or bleeding (9). Black cohosh is contraindicated in individuals with endometriosis or in cases of uterine fibroids (6). In addition, this herb should not be taken during pregnancy as it has been known to stimulate uterine contractions (6). In fact, it is a popular herb used by midwives to induce labor in pregnant women.

Biotin

Purported use: strengthen hair and nails, diabetes, mild depression
Recommended dosage: 2 mg/day. Adequate intake: 30 mcg for adults over 18 years and pregnant women, and 35 mcg for lactating women

Biotin is a B-vitamin that is involved in gluconeogenesis and fatty acid synthesis. Biotin may be sought out by PCOS women for help in improving the common PCOS symptom of alopecia. It has also been suggested that biotin may be helpful for increasing the thickness of nails in those with brittle nails (10). There is also some evidence that diabetes may produce a biotin-deficient state. Biotin has been found to play a role in glucose uptake in skeletal cells and enhancing glucose disposal (10). Research does suggest that a combination of biotin and chromium might lower blood glucose levels in poorly controlled type 2 diabetics. A placebo-controlled, double-blinded, randomized trial examined the effect of chromium picolinate and biotin supplementation on glycemic control in poorly controlled patients with type 2 diabetes mellitus (10). Forty-three subjects with impaired glycemic control were randomized to receive 600 mcg/day of chromium picolinate and 2 mg/day of biotin in addition to oral antihyperglycemic agent therapy for 4 weeks (10). After 4 weeks, significant reductions in glucose and triglycerides were found compared to controls. The researchers suggest that a combination of chromium picolinate and biotin is an effective adjunctive nutritional therapy to people with poorly controlled diabetes with the potential for improving lipid metabolism (10). Biotin alone does not appear to affect glucose or insulin levels in people with type 2 diabetes. No side effects or interactions with any herbs or supplements are known. The use of antibiotics and consuming 2 or more uncooked egg whites per day for several months may affect biotin levels.

Chasteberry
Also known as Vitex angus-castus
Purported use: acne, infertility, hormone regulation, mood swings, progestin effect, stimulates lutenizing hormone
Recommended dosage: 20-40 mg daily

Chasteberry is a popular supplement taken by women with PCOS for its role in regulating hormone levels and possibly improving infertility. Preliminary evidence suggests that chasteberry may have phytoestrogen effects. This herb is proposed to stimulate the pituitary gland and increase levels of lutenizing hormone (LH) and progesterone, increasing the chance of pregnancy in infertile women, however, very few clinical trials involving chasteberry exist. A double-blind, placebo-controlled pilot study examined the effects of a nutritional supplement containing chasteberry on fertility in which 5 of the 15 women in the treatment group became pregnant after 3 months of use (11).

Chasteberry does not work quickly and may take 3-7 months of treatment to promote pregnancy (12). It should not be taken in persons with elevated LH levels (which is commonly seen in PCOS) or in women who are pregnant. There is some evidence that using chasteberry during in vitro fertilization procedures might prevent a pregnancy despite having a viable embryo. In one reported case, a woman undergoing in vitro fertilization began taking chasteberry. She was found to have signs of ovarian hyperstimulation syndrome during her fourth treatment cycle and the embryo did not result in pregnancy (12). Also, because it seems to alter hormone levels, it is not advisable to take chasteberry if you are taking hormone replacement therapy or on birth control medication. Side effects may include GI discomfort, skin rash, headache, diarrhea, nausea, itching, acne, insomnia, weight gain, and irregular menstrual bleeding. Chasteberry may interfere with dopamine antagonist medications (zyprexa, risperdal) (13).

Chromium Picolinate

Purported use: diabetes, food cravings, insulin resistance, and weight loss

Recommended dosage: 500-1000 mcg/day; Adequate intake: 25-30 mcg

Chromium is an essential trace mineral that is involved in carbohydrate metabolism for its role in potentiating insulin (14). Although still not conclusive, supplementation of chromium may be effective in lowering glucose and insulin levels in people with diabetes and insulin resistance (15,16,17). A review of 15 studies on chromium supplementation showed that chromium deficiency results in insulin resistance (17). It was also concluded that insulin resistance due to chromium deficiency can be improved with chromium supplementation (17).

A small study involving three women with PCOS and insulin resistance demonstrated encouraging results with chromium supplementation. These women took 1,000 mcg/day of chromium picolinate for two months, at which time their ability to dispose of glucose improved by 29.5% (18). Another small pilot study found that 200 mcg/day of chromium picolonate improved glucose tolerance in women with PCOS. No affect was found in regards to ovulatory function or hormonal parameters (19). To validate these results, well-controlled randomized trials will need to be conducted. Long-term effects of high doses of chromium are not known. The average American diet is adequate in chromium, however it is theorized that diabetics may be deficient in chromium (14-16). A deficiency in chromium is associated with impaired glucose, insulin, and lipid metabolism (14). Food sources include brewer's yeast, black pepper, mushrooms, broccoli, dried beans, seeds, wine and beer (20). Generally, chromium is well tolerated. Side effects may include headaches, insomnia, sleep disturbances, irritability, and mood changes

(14). Additionally, chromium may cause hypoglycemia in patients taking diabetic medications (20).

Cinnamon Cassia Extract
Purported use: insulin resistance, diabetes, cholesterol, and weight loss
Recommended dosage: 1-6 grams/day

Cinnamon is a popular spice that is believed to make adipose cells more responsive to insulin (21). Studies have shown that cinnamon extract in addition to oral anti-diabetic agents, can improve glucose tolerance in diabetics (22, 23). One study demonstrated that intake of 1-6 grams of cinnamon daily for at least 40 days reduced serum glucose, triglyceride, LDL cholesterol, and total cholesterol levels in people with type 2 diabetes and therefore, may also be beneficial in people with hyperinsulinemia (22). Similar results have also been found in individuals without diabetes (24). Cinnamon seems to work by increasing the phosphorylation of insulin receptors which leads to improved insulin function and improved insulin sensitivity (22). It may also reduce postrprandial insulin response by delaying gastric emptying (24). Since it may lower glucose and insulin levels, careful monitoring of blood sugar levels is important to prevent hypoglycemia. Cinnamon can be sprinkled on cereal, peanut butter sandwiches, oatmeal, and on other foods but must be taken in a capsule form to meet therapeutic dosages.

D-Chiro-inositol
Purposed use: insulin resistance, cholesterol, triglycerides, testosterone-lowering, infertility, hypertension
Recommended dosage: up to 1200 mg/day

D-chiro-inositol is a component of the cellular phospholipid membrane. PCOS clients may try taking it for its many claimed abilities to improve PCOS symptoms. D-chiro-inositol is proposed to decrease serum triglyceride and testosterone levels, and reduce HTN. It is also believed that d-chiro-inositol can induce ovulation by improving insulin sensitivity. It is theorized that clients with insulin resistance, including those with impaired glucose tolerance and type

2 diabetes, might have a d-chiro-inositol deficiency (25). Many clients I have talked with who have tried inositol claim that it promotes the hair growth on their heads and prevents balding. Generally, d-chiro-inositol is well tolerated. It can cause nausea, tiredness, headaches, and dizziness. No interactions with herbs and supplements are known. There is concern, however, that high consumption of d-chiro-inositol might exacerbate bipolar disorder (25).

L-Arginine
Purported use: coronary artery disease, hypertension, cholesterol
Recommended dosage: 6-20 grams daily

L-arginine is an amino acid necessary for protein synthesis. It is found naturally in foods such as red meat, poultry, fish, and dairy products. L-arginine can improve coronary endothelial function and brachial artery endothelium dilation and reduce endothelial cell adhesion in patients with coronary artery disease or hypercholesterolemia, resulting in increased coronary blood flow (26). L-arginine also increases nitric oxide, which causes vasodilation and reduces blood pressure. Side effects include abdominal pain and bloating, diarrhea, and gout (26).

Fenugreek
Also known as Trigonella foenum-graecum or Bird's Foot
Purported use: increase milk production and breast growth, diabetes, insulin resistance
Recommended dosage: 580 or 610 mg 2x/day

Fenugreek is a popular and effective herbal supplement used by nursing mothers to boost milk supply. It may also help with breast development (one cause of insufficient milk production in PCOS women). It is an herbal galactagogue which means it stimulates milk production and it contains some of the same chemicals as metformin and may reduce glucose and insulin levels. The first recorded use of fenugreek is described on an ancient Egyptian papyrus dated to 1500 B.C. Fenugreek seed is commonly used in cooking (27). You can buy fenugreek capsules containing ground seeds at most health food stores. It is also sold in teas known as Mother's Milk which also contains fennel and other herbs reportedly used to boost milk production. Possible side effects of fenugreek when taken by mouth include gas, bloating, and diarrhea. Diabetics should use this herb with caution as it can lower blood glucose levels (27). Pregnant women should not take fenugreek since it may stimulate the uterus, causing contractions (27). There are no apparent side effects in babies whose mothers take the herb. Most mothers will see an increase in milk supply within 24-72 hours (28).

Fish Oil Supplements (Omega-3 Fatty Acids)

Purported use: acne, anti-inflammatory, hyperlipidemia, hypertension, triglycerides, depression, food cravings, hair loss, hormone balance, infertility, insulin resistance, diabetes, and mood swings among many others.

Recommended dosage: currently no recommended amount in the U.S. In Canada the recommended amount is 1-1.5 grams/day. Up to 3 grams per day appears to be well tolerated.

Fatty fish such as herring, kipper, mackerel, menhaden, pilchard, salmon, sardine, and trout contain oils with high amounts of long-chain, polyunsaturated fats called omega-3 fatty acids, specifically eicosapentaenoic acid (EPA) and docosahexaenoic acid (DHA). The body cannot produce omega-3 fatty acids and it is unable to convert omega-6 fatty acids into omega-3 fatty acids. Additionally, omega-3 fatty acids metabolically compete for absorption with omega-6 fatty acids so that a diet that rich in omega-6 fatty acids (the typical Western diet) may be deficient in omega-3 fatty acids. Alpha-linolenic acid (ALA), another omega-3 fatty acid is plant-derived and is slowly converted into EPA and DHA.

Long known for their role in treating mood disorders and depression (29), fish oils containing EPA and DHA may also be used with PCOS to reduce triglyceride levels and aid in regulating hormone levels (30). In fact, many physicians I work with who specialize in treating PCOS have been prescribing a specific fish oil supplement named Lovaza™ (Reliant Pharmaceuticals, Inc.) to their PCOS clients who have hypertriglyceridemia. Lovaza™ contains 460 mg of EPA and

380 mg of DHA in 1 gram capsules and is FDA-approved for treating hypertriglyceridemia (triglyceride levels of 500 mg/dL and above) in conjunction with dietary modifications. Additionally, omega-3 fatty acids have been shown to inhibit platelet aggregation, lower blood pressure, improve lipid levels, and possibly aid in lowering glucose and insulin levels. In 2000, the FDA approved the health claim for labeling omega-3 fatty acids that it is "suggestive, but not conclusive" in reducing the risk of coronary heart disease.

Patients should be advised on ways to regularly incorporate foods rich in the omega-3 fatty acids DHA and EPA into their diet by including at least 2 servings (4 ounces each) of fatty types of fish weekly or take fish oil supplements regularly. There is some concern that fish or fish oil products might be contaminated with toxins or pesticides if the fish were caught in contaminated waters that include mercury or polychlorinated biphenyls (PCBs). Because of this, consumption of farmed salmon which contains higher amounts of mercury than wild salmon, should be limited to no more than 10 times per month. Laboratory analysis of fish oil supplements found no detectable levels of mercury or other toxins in over 20 products tested. However, contaminants including PCBs have been reported in certain brands (31).

Fish oil supplements are generally well tolerated but may cause heartburn, nausea and loose stools in some individuals. Taking them with food may decrease side effects. The FDA concludes that up to 3 grams of EPA and DHA are "Generally Recogonized as Safe (GRAS)." Doses greater than 3 grams per day of fish oil or high dietary intake of fish (greater than 46 grams per day) may inhibit platelet aggregation and cause bleeding. Fish oils do contribute to caloric intake and may cause weight gain if used with an excessive caloric diet (one gram of fat or oil provides 9 kcal). Patients who are allergic to fish or seafood should avoid fish oil supplements

Magnesium
Purported use: diabetes, insulin resistance, hypertension, hyperlipidemia, osteoporosis
Recommended dosage: 600-1000 mg/day; Tolerable upper limit: 350 mg/

day

Magnesium is an essential mineral important in bone structure, fat and protein synthesis, production of ATP and is involved in over 300 different enzyme systems. One study found significantly lower magnesium levels in PCOS patients compared with the controls (32). Magnesium supplementation may be beneficial to women with PCOS due to its ability to reduce insulin, glucose (33), dyslipidemia (33), blood pressure (34), and overall risk of metabolic syndrome (MBS) (33,35).

A higher intake of magnesium is associated with a 31% lower risk of developing MBS in young adults (35) and a 27% lower risk of developing MBS in healthy women (36). Magnesium seems to play a role in regulating glucose levels by influencing the release and activity of insulin (37). It is estimated that 25-38% of individuals with type 2 diabetes have hypomagnesemia and it is suggested that people with low serum magnesium levels are 6-7 times more likely to have MBS than people with normal magnesium levels (26).

A meta-analysis of magnesium supplementation and blood pressure showed a reduction of 4.3 mmHg systolic blood pressure and 2.3 mmHg diastolic blood pressure for each increase of 10 mmol/day of magnesium (34). In addition, individuals with low levels of Vitamin D or parathyroid hormone may also have a magnesium deficiency. Taking magnesium may decrease low-density lipoprotein (LDL) and total cholesterol levels as well as improve high-density lipoprotein (HDL) levels (33,36-38).

Magnesium is found in certain types of fish, whole grains, some fruits, nuts, seeds, legumes, and soy products (33). Magnesium can cause gastrointestinal irritation, nausea, vomiting, and diarrhea. Although rare, larger amounts might cause hypermagnesemia with symptoms including thirst, hypotension, drowsiness, confusion, loss of tendon reflexes, muscle weakness, respiratory depression, cardiac arrhythmias, coma, cardiac arrest, and death (36). High doses of zinc, greater than 142 mg/day, can decrease magnesium absorption as zinc and magnesium compete for transport in the body (36).

St. John's Wort

Also known as Hypericum perforatum
Purported use: mild to moderate depression, anxiety
Recommended dosage: 300-1200 mg/day

St. John's Wort is an herb that has been known for its use in treating mild to moderate depression and anxiety, and may benefit women with PCOS who struggle with these illnesses. In fact, it is the most widely used antidepressant in Germany for its effectiveness in improving mood, decreasing anxiety and improving insomnia among depressed individuals. It is thought to be a selective inhibitor of serotonin, dopamine, and norpepinephrine reuptake in the central nervous system, much like prescribed antidepressants. Overall, St. John's Wort is well tolerated. Adverse effects include photosensitization, headache, nausea, abdominal discomfort, dry mouth, hypertension, and weakness (39). St. John's Wort may cause hypoglycemia in some individuals. Three cases of mania with pre-existing bipolar disorder have been reported (39). Because St. John's Wort is metabolized in the liver by cytochrome P450 system, it can increase or decrease the elimination of many prescription drugs (39). It may decrease the effectiveness of birth control medications. This herb should not be taken while on other herbal supplements, antidepressants or mood stabilizers and should not be used for major depression. St. John's Wort is contraindicated in pregnancy (39).

Saw Palmetto

Also known as Serenoa repens
Purported use: androgen-lowering, anti-inflammatory
Recommended dosage: 160-320 mg/day

Native to North America, saw palmetto is a popular herbal supplement among PCOS women for its proposed anti-androgenic effects. The berries of the saw palmetto plant contain sterols, fatty acids, and flavonoids are believed to inhibit the conversion of testosterone to dihydrotestosterone (DHT) (40). DHT is the hormone in the skin that stimulates hirsutism, contributing to the male pattern hair growth, acne, and alopecia seen in women with PCOS. To date, no studies have been conducted on the effects of saw palmetto on PCOS. The studies that have been conducted have been limited to 6 months, but no adverse effects and no herb-drug interactions have been reported (41,42). Side effects are minor and include dizziness, headaches, and gastrointestinal disturbances (41,42). Patients may have to take it for 6 weeks to see noticeable changes (41). It should not be used while taking oral contraceptives as saw palmetto appears to alter hormone levels (41).

Vanadium
Vanadyl sulfate or vandate
Purported use: insulin resistance, diabetes, hyperlipidemia
Recommended dosage: unkown; Tolerable upper limit: 1.8 mg/day elemental vanadium

Vanadium is a trace mineral non-essential to humans that is believed to increase glucose uptake in muscle cells and improve insulin sensitivity in patients with type 2 diabetes (43-47). However, most clinical trials consist of small sample sizes and are very short in duration (4-6 weeks). Food sources rich in vanadium include shellfish, parsley, mushrooms, wine, and dill seed (48). Note: vanadium may cause renal toxicity and is contraindicated in pregnancy. Side effects include gastrointestinal disturbances such as cramping, diarrhea, and abdominal pain (48) and may not be advisable for women who are also taking metformin. Vanadium may have blood-thinning effects and should not be taken with anticoagulants (49). Other dietary supplements with less side effects than vanadium may be better choices for women with PCOS who are trying to lower their insulin levels.

Vitamin D
Purported use: hypertension, insulin resistance, diabetes, infertility
Recommended dosage: 1,000 IU daily; AI: 200 IU; UL: 2,000 IU/day

It has been suggested that vitamin D deficiency has become an epidemic in our country (50). A deficiency of vitamin D not only causes poor bone mineralization but also has been implicated in numerous chronic diseases including diabetes, heart disease, immunity, various cancers, multiple sclerosis, rheumatoid arthritis, and hypertension (50,51). Vitamin D receptors have now been identified in almost every tissue and cell in the human body, plus the vitamin has been found to be involved in follicle egg maturation and development (52). In fact, in a small trial of 13 women with PCOS who were deficient in vitamin D, normal menstrual cycles resumed within 2 months in 7 of the 9 women who had irregular menstrual cycles when given vitamin D repletion with calcium therapy (52). The authors of the study suggest that abnormalities in calcium homeostasis may be responsible, in part, for the arrested follicular development in women with PCOS and may even contribute to the pathogenesis of the syndrome (52). It has been suggested that vitamin D may play a key role in glucose regulation (51,53,54). Low levels of vitamin D have been negatively correlated with the incidence of type 1 and 2 diabetes (50,51,55).

Many researchers believe the current amount for vitamin D is set too low at 200 IU daily and should be increased. The tolerable upper limit (UL) for Vitamin D is 2,000 IU per day, however, no adverse effects have been found up to 10,000 IU per day (56). Few foods contain vitamin D other than milk fortified with vitamin D, eggs, liver, cereals with vitamin D added, and fatty fish. While skin exposure to the sun provides as much as 80 to 90% of the body's vitamin D, production is limited with the use of sunscreens. The elderly and dark skinned people may be at risk for a vitamin D deficiency as melanin blocks the precursor of active vitamin D in the skin. Obese individuals have a greater chance of lacking vitamin D because it is a fat-soluble vitamin and may not be as bioavailable in high amounts of fat tissue. In fact, obese people may have as much as a 57% reduction in serum vitamin D levels compared to thin individuals, as bioavailability is reduced both by skin synthesis and gastrointestinal absorption (56). Because of this, I usually will recommend my PCOS clients consider taking a vitamin D supplement and have their blood levels checked. Blood levels of vitamin D can be measured by checking 25 hydroxy-vitamin D3 levels and should really be a part of an annual physical examination for all individuals. Optimal levels should be above 20 ng/ml (24). Calcitriol (active vitamin D3) is the most absorbed form of the vitamin. The following are some food sources of vitamin D (57,58):

Food	International Units (IU) Per Serving
Cod liver oil, 1 Tablespoon	1,360
Salmon, 3.5 ounces	360
Tuna fish, canned, 3 ounces	200
Milk, fortified (any type), 8 ounces	98
Cereals, fortified with 10% DV of Vitamin D	40
Egg, 1 whole	20
Cheese, 1 ounce	12

COMPLEMENTARY TREATMENTS FOR PCOS

ACUPUNCTURE

Acupuncture is a form of traditional Chinese medicine that dates back more than 3,000 years and appears to be beneficial in restoring ovulation and increasing the chances of pregnancy in women with PCOS (59). Its drug-free philosophy is based on restoring chi or energy flow within the body. There are believed to be over 2,000 acupuncture points in the body and a blockage of energy at one of these points is thought to be the cause of an illness, pain, or injury. An acupuncturist inserts hair-thin disposable needles to various points in the body, just under the skin to relieve the blockage of energy. Most patients report a heaviness feeling upon insertion and feel very relaxed during the treatment. The needles may be left inserted for up to 45 minutes. Most chronic conditions like PCOS require monthly sessions for best results. Some Western physicians believe that acupuncture works by stimulating the release of endorphins, known as the body's natural pain killers.

Many studies have been conducted throughout the world documenting the success of acupuncture in improving infertility. In one study, 24 women with PCOS who had absent or infrequent periods underwent electro-acupuncture, a form of acupuncture that stimulates electrical currents through the needles. After 10-14 treatments that lasted up to 3 months, 38% of the women experienced regular ovulation (59). Additionally, acupuncture may also improve the success rate of women undergoing in-vitro fertilization (IVF). Forty-three percent of women who received acupuncture before and after undergoing IVF treatments became pregnant compared to 26% of aged-matched women who only did IVF. This shows almost a 50% effective rate of IVF when combined with acupuncture (60). Since IVF is so financially and emotionally taxing, some couples may want to consider the use of acupuncture to increase their chances of conceiving.

OTHER COMPLEMENTARY TREATMENTS

In addition to acupuncture, other forms of complementary treatments may also be beneficial in treating PCOS. Acupressure, reflexology, Reiki, and aromatherapy are all treatments that have been speculated to improve some PCOS symptoms. Tai Chi and yoga are forms of physical activity combined with mindfulness that have also been shown to be benefit women with PCOS.

In summary, the use of dietary supplements is rising in popularity among Americans. Many women with PCOS who are frustrated with their symptoms and medical treatment may turn to dietary supplements instead of, or in conjunction with medications to improve infertility and other symptoms. Therefore, dietitians need to familiarize themselves with dietary supplements that are common among the PCOS community. However, safety is a big concern as dietary supplements are not yet well regulated by the FDA and in most instances, clinical trials are limited in duration and consist of small sample sizes. Therefore, as a dietitian, I am hesitant to recommend the use of any dietary supplement unless sufficient evidence suggests the benefits and safety of its use. Examples of supplements in which insufficient evidence exists include black cohosh, chasteberry, and vanadium.

The most common dietary supplements I recommend to my patients with PCOS are vitamin D, chromium picolinate, cinnamon extract, magnesium, and fish oils. Of course, the recommendation of any supplement should be individualized and given after completing a detailed nutrition assessment where diet intake, supplement, and medication use are assessed. Also, effects of the supplement must be regularly monitored. It is recommended that patients discuss their supplement use with their physicians prior to use. They also need to be educated on potential side effects and the importance of not exceeding recommended dosages. The use of dietary supplements with PCOS is an exciting and important area of study. Dietitians should participate in outcome research for dietary evidence-based guidelines.

REFERENCES

1. Food and Drug Administration. HHS Acts to Reduce Potential Risks of Dietary Supplements Containing Ephedra. February 28, 2003. www.cfsan.fda.gov.

2. Food and Drug Administration. Final Rule for Current Good Manufacturing Practices (CGMPs) for Dietary Supplements, June 22, 2007. www.cfsan.fda.gov.

3. Jacob S, Henriksen EJ, Schiemann AL. Enhancement of glucose disposal in patients with type 2 diabetes by alpha-lipoic acid. *Arzneimittelforschung.* 1995;45:872-874.

4. Packer L, Tritschler HJ, Wessel K. Neuroprotection by the metabolic antioxidant alpah-lipoic acid. *Free Radic Biol Med.* 1997;22 :359-378.

5. Jacob S, Ruus P, Hermann R, Tritschler HJ, Maerker E, Renn W, Augustin HJ, Dietze GJ, Rett K. Oral administration of RAC-alpha-lipoic acid modulates insulin sensitivity in patients with type-2 diabetes mellitus: a placebo-controlled pilot trial. *Free Radic Biol Med.* 1999; 27:309-14.

6. Sarubin Fragakis A. Black Cohosh. In: Sarubin Fragakis A. *The Health Professional's Guide to Popular Dietary Supplements.* 2nd ed. American Dietetic Association; 2003:36-40.

7. Liske E, Hanggi MD, Henneicke-von Zepelin HH, et al.: Physiological investigation of a unique extract of black cohosh (Cimicifugae racemosae rhizoma): a 6-month clinical study demonstrates no systemic estrogenic effect. *Journal of Women's Health & Gender-Based Medicine.* 2002;11: 163-174.

8. Stoll W: Phytotherapy influences atrophic vaginal epithelium:

Double-blind study of Cimicifuga vs. estrogenic substances (in German). *Therapeutikon.* 1987;1:23-31.

9. Gruenwald J. Standardized black cohosh (Cimicifuga) extract clinical monograph. *Quarterly Review of Natural Medicine* (Summer). 1998;117-125.

10. Singer GM, Geohas J. The effect of chromium picolinate and biotin supplementation on glycemic control in poorly controlled patients with type 2 diabetes mellitus: a placebo-controlled, double-blinded, randomized trial. *Diabetes Technol Ther.* 2006; 8:636-43.

11. Westphal LM, Polan ML, Trant AS, Mooney SB. A nutritional supplement for improving fertility in women: a pilot study. *J Reprod Med.* 2004;49:289-93.

12. Chasteberry. Natural Medicines Comprehensive Database Web site. Accessed on December 28, 2006.

13. Roemheld-Hamm B. Chasteberry. *Am Fam Physician.* 2005; 72:821-4.

14. A scientific review: the role of chromium in insulin resistance. *Diabetes Educ.* 2004; Suppl:2-14.

15. Vladeva SV, Terzieva DD, Arabadjiiska DT. Effect of chromium on the insulin resistance in patients with type II diabetes mellitus. *Folia Med* (Plovdiv). 2005;47:59-62.

16. Anderson RA, Cheng N, Bryden NA, et al. Elevated intakes of supplemental chromium improve glucose and insulin variables in individuals with type II diabetes. *Diabetes.* 1997;46:1786-1791.

17. Mertz W. Chromium in human nutrition: a review. *J Nutr.* 1993;123:626-633.

18. Lydic ML, McNurlan M, Komaroff E, et al. Effects of chromium supplementation on insulin sensitivity and reproductive function in polycystic ovarian syndrome: A pilot study. *Fertility and Sterility.* 2003;80:45-46(abstract).

19. Lucidi R, Thyer A, Easton C, Holden A. Effect of chromium supplementation on insulin resistance and ovarian and menstrual cyclicity in women with polycystic ovary syndrome. *Fertility and Sterility.* 2005;84(6):1755-1757.

20. Sarubin Fragakis A. Chromium. In: Sarubin Fragakis A *The Health Professional's Guide to Popular Dietary Supplements.* 2nd ed. American Dietetic Association; 2003:85-94.

21. Anderson, R.A. 2005. Polyphenols from cinnamon increase insulin

sensitivity: Functional and clinical aspects [abstract]. *Dietary Antioxidants, Trace Elements, Vitamins and Polyphenols.* 2005;4:154.

22. Khan A, Safdar M, Khan MMA, et al. Cinnamon improves glucose and lipids of people with type 2 diabetes. *Diabetes Care.* 2003;26:3215-3218.

23. Mang B, Wolters M, Schmitt B, Kelb K, Lichtinghagen R, Stichtenoth DO, Hahn A. Effects of a cinnamon extract on plasma glucose, HbA, and serum lipids in diabetes mellitus type 2. *Eur J Clin Invest.* 2006;36:340-4.

24. Hlebowicz J, Darwiche G, Bjorgell O, Olof L. Effect of cinnamon on postprandial blood glucose, gastric emptying, and satiety in healthy subjects. *Amer J Clin Nutr.* 2007;85(6):1552-1556.

25. d-chiro-inositol. Natural Medicines Comprehensive Database Web site. Accessed on January 2, 2007.

26. Sarubin Fragakis A. Arginine. In: Sarubin Fragakis A. *The Health Professional's Guide to Popular Dietary Supplements.* 2nd ed. American Dietetic Association; 2003:20-30.

27. Fenugreek. Natural Medicines Comprehensive Database Web site. Accessed on January 2, 2007

28. Marasco L, Marmet C, Shell E. Polycystic Ovary Syndrome: A connection to insufficient milk supply? *Journal of Human Lactation.* 2000;16(2):143-148.

29. Parker G, Gibson NA, Brotchie H, et al. Omega-3 fatty acids and mood disorders. *Amer J Psych.* 2006;163:969-980.

30. Bhathena SJ. Relationship between fatty acids and the endocrine system. *Biofactors.* 2000;13:35-9.

31. Fish Oils. Natural Medicines Comprehensive Database Web site. Accessed on January 12, 2007.

32. Muneyyirci-Delale, O et al, Divalent cations in women with PCOS: implications for cardiovascular disease. *Gynecol Endocrinol.* 2001;15(3):198-201.

33. Feldeisen S, Tucker K. Nutritional stratagies in the prevention and treatment of metabolic syndrome. *Appl Physiol Nutr Metabolism* 2007;32:46-60.

34. Jee SH, Miller ER, Guallar E, Sing VK, Appel LJ, Klag MJ. The effect of magnesium supplementation on blood pressure: a meta-analysis of randomized clinical trials. *Am J Hypertens.* 2002;14:691-696.

35. He K, Liu K, Daviglus ML, Morris SJ, Loria CM. Magnesium intake and incidence of metabolic syndrome among young adults. *Circulation.* 2006;113:1675-1682.

36. Magnesium. Natural Medicines Comprehensive Database Web site. Accessed on December 29, 2006.

37. Kobrin SM, Goldfarb S. Magnesium Deficiency. *Semin Nephrol.* 1990;10:525-35.

38. Sarubin Fragakis A. Magnesium. In: Sarubin Fragakis A. *The Health Professional's Guide to Popular Dietary Supplements.* 2nd ed. American Dietetic Association; 2003:280-291.

39. St. John's Wort. Natural Medicines Comprehensive Database Web site. Accessed on December 29, 2006.

40. Niederprum HJ, Schweikert HU, Zanker KS. Testosterone 5a-reductase inhibition by free fatty acids from sabal serrulata fruits. *Phytomedicine.* 1994;1:127-133.

41. Saw Palmetto. Natural Medicines Comprehensive Database Web site. Accessed on January 29, 2007.

42. Sarubin Fragakis A. Saw Palmetto. In: Sarubin Fragakis A. *The Health Professional's Guide to Popular Dietary Supplements.* 2nd ed. American Dietetic Association; 2003:350-353.

43. Wang J, Yuen VG, McNeill JH. Effect of vanadium on insulin sensitivity and appetite. *Metabolism.* 2001;50(6):667-73.

44. Cusi K, Cukier S, DeFronzo RA, Torres M, Puchulu FM, Redondo JC. Vanadyl sulfate improves hepatic and muscle insulin sensitivity in type 2 diabetes. *J Clin Endocrinol Metab.* 2001;86(3):1410-7.

45. Goldfine AB, Patti ME, Zuberi L, Goldstein BJ, LeBlanc R, Landaker EJ, Jiang ZY, Willsky GR, Kahn CR. Metabolic effects of vanadyl sulfate in humans with non-insulin-dependent diabetes mellitus: in vivo and in vitro studies. *Metabolism.* 2000;49(3):400-10.

46. Cam MC, Brownsey RW, McNeill JH. Mechanisms of vanadium action: insulin-mimetic or insulin-enhancing agent? *Can J Physiol Pharmacol.* 2000;78(10):829-47.

47. Halberstam M, cohen N, Shlimovich P, et al. Oral vanadyl sulfate improves insulin sensitivity in NIDDM but not in obese nondiabeteic subjects. *Diabetes.* 1996;45:659-666.

48. Sarubin Fragakis A. Vanadium. In: Sarubin Fragakis A. *The Health Professional's Guide to Popular Dietary Supplements.* 2nd ed. American

Dietetic Association; 2003:387-392.

49. Vanadium. Natural Medicines Comprehensive Database Web site. Accessed on January 29, 2007.

50. Holick MF. Vitamin D: importance in the prevention of cancers, type 1 diabetes, heart disease, and osteoporosis. *Am J Clin Nutr.* 2004;79(3):362-71.

51. Lips P. Vitamin D physiology. *Prog Biophys Mol Biol.* 2006;(92)1:4-8.

52. Thys-Jacobs S, Donovan D, Papadopoulos A, Sarrel P, Bilezikian JP. Vitamin D and calcium dysregulation in the polycystic ovarian syndrome. *Steroids.* 1999;64(6):430-5.

53. Harkness LS, Bonny AE. Calcium and vitamin D status in the adolescent: key roles for bone, body weight, glucose tolerance, and estrogen biosynthesis. *J Pediatr Adolesc Gynecol.* 2005;18(5):305-11.

54. Chiu KC, et al. Hypovitaminosis D is associated with insulin resistance and beta cell dysfunction. *Am J Clin Nutr.* 2004;79:820-25.

55. Pittas AG, Dawson-Hughes B, Li T, Van Dam RM, Willett WC, Manson JE, Hu FB. Vitamin D and calcium intake in relation to type 2 diabetes in women. *Diabetes Care.* 2006;29(3):650-6.

56. Vitamin D. Natural Medicines Comprehensive Database Web site. Accessed on January 20, 2007.

57. *J P. Bowes and Church's Food Values of Portions Commonly Used.* 17th ed. Philadelphia, PA: Lippincot-Raven; 1998.

58. U.S. Department of Agriculture, Agricultural Research Service. 2003. USDA Nutrient Database for Standard Reference, Release 16. Nutrient Data Laboratory Home Page, http://www.nal.usda.gov/fnic/foodcomponline.

59. Stener-Victorin E et al. Effects of electro-acupuncture on anovulation in women with polycystic ovary syndrome. *Acta Obstet Gynecol Scand.* 2000;79(3):180-8.

60. Paulus, WE. Influence of acupuncture on the pregnancy rate in patients who undergo assisted reproduction therapy. *Fertility and Sterility.* 2002; 77(4):721-724.

CHAPTER 6

PCOS IN ADOLESCENCE

Sara was a 17-year-old who had difficulties managing her weight since entering puberty at an early age. She seemed to crave carbohydrates "all the time," even after eating dinner, and complained that her weight had been increasing at a rate of 1 to 2 pounds per month over the past year. Sara had recently seen a dermatologist for acne on her chin; previously she had no acne problem. She also had recently visited her primary care physician (PCP) for dizziness, feeling shaky, and irregular menses. Her PCP started her on a birth control pill to regulate her periods and diagnosed Sara with hypoglycemia, encouraging her to follow a South Beach-type diet to control her blood sugar and help her lose weight. Nine years later, at age 26, Sara saw an endocrinologist because she could not lose weight, despite her efforts, and because she was experiencing severe hypoglycemia and had elevated serum triglycerides. Sara was diagnosed with polycystic ovarian syndrome (PCOS).

Adolescence is the most vulnerable and influential stage of PCOS. It is usually in adolescence when symptoms of PCOS first start to present themselves in young women. It is during this period when changes can be made in regards to diet and lifestyle that could prevent the worsening of symptoms later in life and prevent the onset of many health complications. Many of the symptoms young women first experience such as acne, irregular menses, hair loss, and weight gain, are common conditions "normally" experienced during adolescence and can easily be overlooked. In fact, due to the vast array of symptoms and because not every woman may recognize them, PCOS can be very difficult to diagnose. Dietitians, because of their unique role in developing an ongoing relationship with their adolescent patients, may be able to help connect the pieces of the puzzle by recognizing the symptoms patients experience and encourage further diagnostic testing.

THE IMPORTANCE OF EARLY RECOGNITION AND TREATMENT OF ADOLESCENTS WITH POLYCYSTIC OVARY SYNDROME

Because PCOS is linked to the development of chronic diseases (i.e., type 2 diabetes, heart disease, hypertension, and endometrial cancer) later in life, early recognition and treatment is critical to prevent the development of these conditions. Furthermore, since most adult women with PCOS are not diagnosed until after seeking help with infertility, early detection in adolescence could prevent financial and emotional hardships in adulthood.

There is no question that PCOS worsens with age. Adult women with PCOS have a 5-10 times greater chance of developing type 2 diabetes (T2DM) than do women without PCOS (1) and the progression starts early. Research shows that obese PCOS adolescents have one-half the peripheral tissue insulin sensitivity than that of obese adolescents without PCOS (2). Also, it has been shown that adolescent girls with PCOS are at an increased risk for metabolic syndrome compared to adolescent girls in the general population (3). Additionally, being obese may increase the risk for complications during pregnancy such as gestational diabetes, pre-eclampsia, premature labor, miscarriage, or still birth. Therefore, early intervention is imperative to prevent these conditions by establishing a lifetime pattern of physical activity and healthful eating (4).

Just as important, many of the signs and symptoms of PCOS can be very detrimental to a young woman's body image. The most notable of these are weight gain, excessive hair growth on the face and body, "dirty looking" patches on skin (acanthosis nigricans, clinical markers of hyperinsulinemia) and acne. Such clinical features can have a significant impact on the emotional health of an adolescent at a time when self image is developing and social acceptance is so valued. Depression is common among adolescent girls with PCOS (4,5), either due to hormonal imbalances or struggles with body image. Moreover, attempts at weight loss can lead to distorted eating practices or eating disorders. In fact, about one-third of PCOS women have abnormal eating patterns and 6% are bulimic (6). Some young woman with PCOS may feel that that having high levels of testosterone and excess weight around their mid-section makes them less feminine and more masculine. They may even try and "prove" their femininity by being sexually promiscuous, often engaging in unprotected sex to become pregnant, the ultimate sign of femininity (4,7).

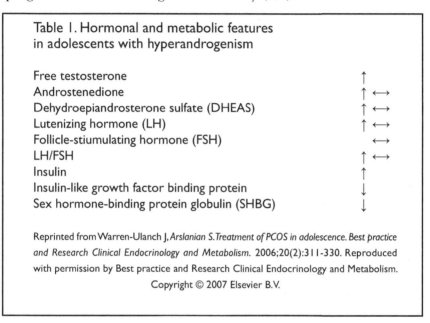

Table 1. Hormonal and metabolic features in adolescents with hyperandrogenism

Free testosterone	↑
Androstenedione	↑ ⟷
Dehydroepiandrosterone sulfate (DHEAS)	↑ ⟷
Lutenizing hormone (LH)	↑ ⟷
Follicle-stiumulating hormone (FSH)	⟷
LH/FSH	↑ ⟷
Insulin	↑
Insulin-like growth factor binding protein	↓
Sex hormone-binding protein globulin (SHBG)	↓

Reprinted from Warren-Ulanch J, Arslanian S. Treatment of PCOS in adolescence. Best practice and Research Clinical Endocrinology and Metabolism. 2006;20(2):311-330. Reproduced with permission by Best practice and Research Clinical Endocrinology and Metabolism. Copyright © 2007 Elsevier B.V.

DIAGNOSING POLYCYSTIC OVARY SYNDROME IN ADOLESCENTS

There has been increasing awareness of the existence of PCOS in adolescents, yet there remains a knowledge gap when it comes to making an accurate diagnosis. According to current consensus, diagnosis of PCOS is made if two of the following three criteria are present (8):

1. Oligomenorrhea (period intervals of > 40 days) or amenorrhea

2. Clinical and/or biochemical signs of hyperandrogenism

3. Polycystic ovaries on an ultrasound, with exclusion of other causes

Unfortunately, these criteria were developed for the adult woman with PCOS and did not take the adolescent population into consideration. This is particularly important considering that symptoms of anovulation and hyperandrogenism may vary and appear at different ages among adolescents, if appearing at all. In fact, it has even been suggested that girls as young as 3 years can start to show signs of the clinical manifestations of PCOS (9). Therefore, the current diagnostic criteria for PCOS may not be entirely appropriate for diagnosing PCOS in adolescents. Table 1 shows the typical metabolic and reproductive features in adolescents with hyperandrogenism.

INSULIN RESISTANCE

Currently, insulin resistance is not part of the diagnostic criteria for PCOS, but is a classic feature of the syndrome. Acanthosis nigricans (raised, dark, velvety patches of skin usually found behind the neck, armpits, or knuckles) are clinical signs of elevated insulin levels (4). Dry and rough elbows, skin tags (also seen with obesity), and "rings" or lines in the skin around the neck may be seen as well. In fair skinned women, some of these signs may be difficult to spot. There is a correlation between an increase in BMI and severity of insulin resistance. In the case of PCOS, excess weight found around the midsection with an excess waist-to-hip ratio (> .85) is attributed to insulin resistance (7). The accumulation of weight around the abdominal area can be very upsetting and frustrating to young women with PCOS as it is very difficult to lose and sets them apart from their peers. A few of my adolescent patients (and some adults) have referred to the excess weight as a "spare tire" or "inner tube" around their waist. One teenager even named her extra weight, referring to it as Maurice.

According to Dr. Katherine Sherif, at Drexel University's Center for Women's Health and The PCOS Program, insulin resistance acts as an appetite stimulant. "When cells are starved of glucose, as in the case of insulin resistance, they only want more energy, thus stimulating appetite to meet those needs (10)." Another problem with having elevated insulin levels is hypoglycemia, which often results in carbohydrate cravings and can contribute to binge eating.

Insulin levels can be detected by a fasting insulin level or as part of an oral glucose tolerance test (OGTT). Fasting glucose levels should also be obtained regularly to screen for diabetes but usually presents as normal in young women with PCOS until later in life, despite elevated insulin levels. In adult women, a fasting glucose-to-insulin ratio less than 4.5 has been shown to be an indicator of insulin resistance (11).

ANOVULATORY SYMPTOMS

Anovulatory symptoms range and may be classified as amenorrhea (no periods at all), oligomenorrhea (≤ 6 cycles per year or > 40 day cycles), very light flow, or dysfunctional uterine bleeding with heavy and painful periods (7,12). Although menstrual disturbances are perhaps the hallmark feature physicians look for when diagnosing PCOS, it is actually very common for a young woman to experience some form of menstrual disturbances as a natural part of puberty. In fact, by the third year after menarche, 59% of cycles will remain anovulatory in normal females (13). Therefore, the diagnostic criteria of anovulation or oligoamenorrhea may not always be appropriate in diagnosing adolescents with PCOS.

Unfortunately, many teenagers with oligomenorrhea do not seek help from their physician and all too often, those that do may just be prescribed oral contraceptives to regulate menstrual function, instead of being recommended for further endocrine evaluation (4).

HYPERANDROGENISM

Hyperandrogenism is classified by acne, hirsutism (dark, coarse hairs on the face, back abdomen, inner thighs or chest) and male-pattern baldness or hair thinning (12). Acne might be a more sensitive sign of androgen excess than hirsutism in adolescents because of the time it takes to grow hair (12). Elevated androgen levels may in fact be the most reliable indicator of PCOS in the pediatric or adolescent population, since 66% of PCOS adolescents will experience some signs of it (7). However, just like the other symptoms of PCOS, signs of excess androgens may not appear in all adolescents, or may appear at different stages of development with different degrees of severity (7). Hyperandrogenism has been proposed to influence intra-abdominal fat as androgen receptors have been located on adipocytes, contributing to the weight loss difficulties women with PCOS(14). In addition, hyperandrogenism has been suggested as an independent risk factor for metabolic syndrome in PCOS (3), supporting the need for early detection and intervention during adolescence.

EARLY PUBERTY

One of the first signs of PCOS may be premature pubarche defined as the presence of pubic hair before the age of 8 and is associated with a history of low birth weight (LBW) (14,15). In fact, researchers have found an increased frequency of menstrual dysfunction and hyperandrogenism among girls with precocious pubarche who were born LBW (16). Premature pubarche is a risk factor for hyperinsulinemia and dyslipidemia in adolescence (9). Sex hormone-binding protein globulin (SHBG) appears to be decreased in girls with premature pubarche as well (16). It appears that African American and Caribbean Hispanic girls are more prone to developing premature pubarche and PCOS due to earlier and higher levels of androgens (9). Therefore, these populations should be monitored closely throughout adolescence and early adulthood for signs of persistent insulin resistance and hyperandrogenism that may indicate PCOS (9).

POLYCYSTIC OVARIES

According to Salmi et al, "not all women with polycystic ovaries have PCOS, and not all women with PCOS have polycystic ovaries" (4). It is estimated that up to 25% of women without PCOS have cysts around their ovaries, as shown upon an ultrasound. Therefore, despite the syndrome's name, the presence of cysts alone is not sufficient for the diagnosis (4). It is important to keep in mind that the cysts are not a cause of PCOS but rather a result of hormonal imbalances affecting the ovary; they are not usually painful or dangerous (12). The ultrasound criteria for a PCOS diagnosis includes the presence of ≥ 10 folliciles, 2 to 9 mm in diameter and located peripherally on at least one ovary, increasing the size of the ovary (8). Polycystic-appearing ovaries alone are not sufficient criteria to make the diagnosis of PCOS as ovarian cysts may be part of other conditions such as congenital adrenal hyperplasia, hypothalamic amenorrhea, and hyperprolactinemia or a normal part of puberty (9,12).

FAMILY HISTORY

Family history is another risk factor for PCOS. First-degree relatives of women with PCOS typically have higher levels of androgens. In one study, 35% of mothers and 40% of sisters of affected women also had PCOS (17). Therefore, if PCOS does run in the family, especially if a mother or sister has it, early testing for the diagnosis is warranted. Alternatively, if a teen is diagnosed with PCOS, it is also important to screen any of her sisters for it, keeping in mind that symptoms with PCOS vary and appear at different stages of adolescence.

EPILEPSY AND PCOS

Interestingly, it does appear that there is an increased risk of PCOS in women with epilepsy. One study showed that 26% of women with epilepsy also had PCOS. It is hypothesized that there may be a dysfunction of the hypothalamus in regards to reproductive function among epileptics or that valproic acid, used in the treatment of epilepsy, may cause PCOS (18). Since the prevalence of PCOS is three to five times higher than normal in epileptic women, it is suggested that this population be screened early for PCOS and other endocrine disorders (4).

THE DIETITIAN AS DETECTIVE

As dietitians, we have a unique advantage in the ability to recognize PCOS among our adolescent patients because we see patients longer and more frequently. The relationship established with our patients can give us a better sense of their dietary intake, activity levels, cravings, hunger patterns, as well as their feelings toward food and weight. We also have the ability to track patients' symptoms on a more regular basis than perhaps other health professionals. Most commonly, an adolescent, her parents, or physician will seek advice from a dietitian for help in managing her weight without knowing she has PCOS.

The initial nutrition assessment is an optimal time to quickly screen any female adolescent patient, regardless of her weight status, for possible signs of PCOS. I have found the best time to do this is while inquiring about any medical concerns. I will routinely ask some probing questions pertaining to oligomenorrhea and hirsutism such as "tell me what your periods are like. Are they heavy, irregular, absent?" and "can you tell me about any excessive body hair that you experience?" If any of the answers to the above questions are yes, and if the patient does have some irregularity to her periods (especially if they are non-existent), or has excess weight around her mid-section with difficulties losing weight, I will usually probe further asking the patient if she has ever heard of PCOS or if someone in the family has it. Additionally, I will ask other screening questions like "tell me about any foods that you typically crave" or "do you ever experience low blood sugar?" See Chapter 4 for questions to ask a patient suspected of PCOS. Additionally, Table 2 lists common indicators of PCOS among adolescents.

Table 2. Common indicators of PCOS among adolescents

Irregular, absent, or heavy menses
Excessive abdominal weight
Significant weight gain without changes to diet or exercise
Difficulties losing weight despite efforts
Excess facial hair or hair on other body areas
Acne
Skin tags
Hair loss from head
Intense carbohydrate cravings
Dark or "dirty-looking" patches on skin

Sometimes simply asking a patient if she was ever told that she had abnormal lab results can uncover possible signs of PCOS. I once saw a 15 year-old whom I suspected had PCOS because of her struggles with weight, acne, and irregular periods. When I asked her this question, she revealed she had once been told, prior to receiving birth control pills to regulate her periods, that she had high testosterone levels, but she had never been diagnosed with PCOS.

If PCOS is suspected, it is imperative that the dietitian refer her patient to a suitable physician knowledgeable in PCOS for diagnosis and treatment and to rule out any other possible medical conditions. The physician may be a reproductive endocrinologist, endocrinologist, gynecologist, or pediatrician. When recommending that the patient seek medical evaluation for PCOS I always give her or her parents a list of recommended lab tests the physician should run to diagnosis PCOS, which includes the hormones listed in table 1. I also encourage patients to ask when scheduling the appointment if the physician is familiar in treating PCOS. It is very surprising how many physicians are unsure about what lab tests to run or do not have adequate knowledge in the area. Both The Polycystic Ovary Association (www.PCOsupport.org) and Project PCOS (www.project-PCOS.org) provide listings of physicians by state. Unfortunately, most adult women with PCOS usually have a story to tell about how they finally got diagnosed after seeing numerous doctors throughout their lives, all of whom overlooked their condition. For this reason, I also recommend that the patient receive a copy of her lab results for her own records, so that she can know what labs were tested. Patients should always trust their instincts and get a second or third opinion if not satisfied with what they were told.

TREATMENT OF POLYCYSTIC OVARY SYNDROME IN ADOLESCENTS

There is much uncertainty regarding proper treatment of PCOS in adolescents. Adult symptoms of PCOS are known to be alleviated by diet, exercise, weight loss, and androgen or insulin-lowering medications (19). However, many of these medications have not been proven to be safe over the long-term for adolescents, and require compliance. Adolescents are more concerned about results "now" and less concerned about improving health in the long run. Their reasons for seeking medical care are that they want to lose weight and improve their dermatological symptoms (i.e., acne, acanthosis nigricans, stretch marks). For some, food has become a control tactic used to set boundaries with parents. Therefore, treatment of an adolescent with PCOS, often requires a multidisciplinary approach involving a pediatrician, dermatologist, endocrinologist, nutritionist, psychiatrist, psychologist, or even a family therapist.

The main goals of treatment for an adolescent with PCOS are to regulate menstrual function, reduce androgen and insulin levels, improve dermatological symptoms, and stabilize or reduce weight.

Treatment goals also need to consider the importance of preventing long-term complications. Treatment is aimed at reducing insulin levels, as it tends to cause a reduction in androgen levels and regulates menses (4,12). Weight loss has been shown to be beneficial in improving metabolic and reproductive parameters in adult women with PCOS, yet is difficult for women with PCOS to achieve. Both from personal experience and from that of my patients, lowering of insulin and androgen levels can lead to some weight loss even without caloric restriction but may take months to see improvements. Therefore, changes in eating and activity patterns will need to be maintained long-term for significant weight loss to occur.

INSULIN SENSITIZERS

Although not yet approved by the Food and Drug Administration (FDA) for its use among individuals with PCOS, metformin (glucophage®, Bristol-Myers Squibb Co.) is the most common medication prescribed for PCOS and its benefits continue to be demonstrated. In addition to improving insulin sensitivity and glucose metabolism, metformin can also ameliorate hyperandrogenism, restore menstrual function and induce ovulation (20). Teenagers with PCOS may benefit more from the use of metformin. Higher success rates have been found in adolescents in regards to normalizing menses and decreasing hirsutism than adults (16,20,-22). In addition, metformin has also been demonstrated to help lower total cholesterol, LDL cholesterol, and triglyceride levels in adolescents with PCOS (16,20). The use of this medication is life long, as discontinuation of metformin therapy has been shown to have renewed progression of PCOS symptoms within 6 months (16). Dosage may range from 1,500-3,000 mg per day. The most common side effects are gastrointestinal issues, most notably diarrhea. This, along with the disadvantage of a large pill size making swallowing difficult, may cause an adolescent to stop taking metformin or take it inconsistently. Lactic acidosis is a rare side effect.

Investigators have recently studied the effects of metformin on prepubertal nonobese girls to stop the progression of PCOS. In their study, 33 LBW prepubertal girls (Tanner Stage 1 of breast development) (16), were randomized to remain untreated or to be treated with metformin (425 mg) once daily at dinner time for 6 months. Fasting blood glucose and serum insulin, Sex hormone-binding protein globulin (SHBG), dehydroepiandrosterone sulfate (DHEAS), testosterone, and lipid profile were assessed at 0 and 6 months, as was body composition. At baseline, both groups showed reduced serum SHBG, increased androgen levels, and abnormal lipid levels, supporting the theory of LBW on the pathogenesis of PCOS and also the long-term cardiovascular disease risk associated with PCOS. The group that was not treated with metformin showed a worsening of assessed lab values at 6 months, including increased body fat. In contrast, the metformin-treated group at 6 months, showed improvements toward normal reference ranges for all parameters. This suggests that treatment with metformin may be used to delay or prevent the onset of PCOS in high risk girls who have a combined history of LBW and premature pubarche (16). The investigators stress that future studies are needed to address the use of metformin in preventing PCOS as well as the safety of longer-term metformin therapy use before puberty, including its possible effects on pubertal growth and development (16). However, the possibility that PCOS may be prevented by medication is certainly encouraging.

When working with an adolescent who takes metformin, it is important to let them know in advance that they need to take the medication with food and that they most likely will be experiencing diarrhea for the first several weeks as their body adjusts to the medication and that it subsides in most individuals. Pill size varies depending on dosage. An extended release version of metformin is available and may have less gastrointestinal side effects.

Thiazolidenediones (TZDs) are other insulin sensitizers such as avandia® (rosiglitazone, GlaxoSmithKline) or actos® (pioglitazone, Takeda Pharmaceuticals North America, Inc.) that can be used alone or in conjunction with metformin to improve insulin sensitivity, reduce androgen levels and hirstuism (and are a much smaller pill size) (23). Whereas metformin works to inhibit hepatic glucose production and increase peripheral insulin sensitivity, TZDs work at the peripheral or cellular level to increase insulin sensitivity (24). Therefore, some patients who do not see reduced insulin levels while taking metformin and making changes to her diet and exercise patterns may find that the addition of a TZD will be more effective (24). However, safety of this class of medications among adolescents is not extensive and may cause hepatotoxicity as well as some initial weight gain (4). Most recently, the FDA issued a safety alert on avadia. This was out of concern of increased risk of heart attacks and heart-related deaths in patients taking avandia. (25). To date, data is still being analyzed by the FDA Advisory Committee. Patients who take avandia are asked to contact their physician about the use of this medication.

ORAL CONTRACEPTIVES

Oral contraceptives (OCPs) may be used among adolescents to regulate menstrual function and hormone levels, as well as decrease acne and hirsutism (4). These may be used on their own or in conjunction with metformin and other medications. They may also be beneficial in increasing bone density, reducing the risk of endo-metrial and ovarian cancer, and preventing anemia (26). Side effects, however, include possible weight gain and increases in triglyceride and cholesterol levels (4) which are not ideal, considering the PCOS population is at an increased risk for obesity and dyslipidemia. In addition, some recent studies have suggested that certain OCPs can actually decrease insulin sensitivity, thus aggravating impaired glucose metabolism in women who have PCOS (27), but more research is needed. If a PCOS adolescent does decide to take OCPs, it is impor-tant that she have regular blood work done to monitor her triglyceride and lipid levels. In addition to monitoring caloric intake, periodic weight checks may be needed to identify possible weight gain.

ANTIANDROGEN THERAPY

Acne and hirsutism can have a significant effect on the body image of a teen with PCOS. Androgen-lowering medications such as spironolactone or flutamide may be prescribed to decrease derma-tological symptoms of hair loss and unwanted facial hair (4) and should be initiated early to prevent significant hair growth which can be longer and more difficult to remove (12). However, none of these medications are approved for the treatment of hirsutism by the FDA and most clinical trials evaluating the safety and efficacy of these drugs among adolescents are limited; there may also be unwanted side effects. Spironolactone should not be taken by women who may become pregnant since it has been linked to birth defects (12). Young women prescribed these medications should be educated that it may take 6 months or longer to see improvement (9). Other forms of hair removal such as shaving, electrolysis, and laser therapy may be safer and faster alternatives to medications.

DIETARY MANAGEMENT FOR POLYCYSTIC OVARY SYNDROME IN ADOLESCENCE

The preferred and most effective method of treatment for PCOS is lifestyle modification (4). Studies are lacking on the proper diet recommendations for adolescents with PCOS; the studies that are available are conflicting. Some studies suggest following a low carbohydrate diet while others suggest a low-glycemic index diet to manage insulin levels (28). Due to elevated insulin levels, women with PCOS tend to crave carbohydrates more than someone without PCOS (29). Therefore, some adolescents may find that severely limiting carbohydrates may be too difficult to follow and could contribute to binge eating and weight gain in the long-run.

To date, no study has proven one diet composition to be superior to another in treating PCOS. Weight loss seems to improve all metabolic and reproductive parameters in PCOS, yet is difficult for most women to achieve. The most beneficial diet for adolescents with PCOS is one that improves insulin sensitivity and dyslipidemia. Therefore, the diet recommendations I advise for adolescents with PCOS is the same as for adult women with the syndrome: a low-saturated fat and lower carbohydrate intake, predominantly from whole grains (28). Emphasis should be on consuming lean protein sources and unsaturated fats, particularly omega-3 fatty acids. The importance of eating often (every 3-5 hours) and including protein with meals and snacks to help manage blood sugar levels and prevent hypoglycemia, needs to be stressed to the adolescent who, like the majority of adolescents, tend to skip meals or wait long periods between eating. Sometimes my adolescent patients will request a note from me or their physician allowing them to have food in school due to medical necessity. This can be beneficial considering that for some teenagers, lunch time is at 10 a.m.! More specific information regarding medical nutrition therapy for PCOS can be found in Chapters 3 and 4. Additionally, sample meal plans using these recommendations can be found in the appendix.

Some teenagers prefer to take nutritional supplements in hopes of improving their PCOS symptoms without medications. Others may decide to try nutritional supplements as an adjunct to their current medical treatment. However, the use of nutritional supplements among adolescents is not clearly understood. For this reason, I am hesitant to recommend any supplements to teenagers except the ones that have the lowest documented side effects and are perhaps the most beneficial to them. These typically include vitamin D, cinnamon extract, fish oils, and chromium picolonate. Of course, it is important for patients to consult their doctors prior to taking any nutritional supplement. Even then, careful monitoring for potential side effects or drug-nutrient interactions is warranted.

OTHER FACTORS TO CONSIDER

Evidence suggests that a moderate weight loss of 5-7% of total body weight may significantly improve all symptoms of PCOS in adults and adolescents, menstrual function and insulin sensitivity (4, 28). Yet, it can be difficult for teens to lose weight while having hyperinsulinemia and hyperandrogensim (9). Furthermore, dieting in adolescence is associated with weight gain later in life and increases the risk of developing an eating disorder (30). For these reasons, more emphasis should be placed on improving the health of adolescents by encouraging a healthy approach to eating and exercise rather than focusing on weight loss. When at all possible, the dietitian should refrain from using calories with their teen patients and should avoid classifying foods as "good" or "bad."

Because of the higher risk of distorted eating and eating disorders among the PCOS population (5, 32), dietitians need to properly screen adolescent clients for abnormal eating behaviors and attitudes toward food and weight. If distorted eating or an eating disorder is suspected, treatment should be aimed at normalizing eating patterns before recommending changes to eating or activity levels. More information on treating eating disorders in PCOS can be found in Chapter

8.

Dietitians will need to take an encouraging, empathetic, and supportive approach when counseling teenagers with PCOS. They need to validate patients that the weight they gained was due to hormonal imbalances and not their fault. Patients need to know that they are not alone in their struggles with PCOS symptoms. Many adolescent patients are already concerned about infertility at a young age and need to be reassured that it is quite possible that they will have no problems conceiving a child. Educating them that improvements in eating and activity patterns are ways to improve fertility may be helpful in encouraging adolescents to implement changes.

Adolescents need to understand in simplified terms the pathophysiology of PCOS and the connections to their symptoms. They will also need to be educated on insulin resistance and why it is so important to make changes in their eating and activity patterns now to prevent further complications. Educating patients on how different foods affect their insulin levels may be particularly helpful. For example, white bread versus whole wheat bread or whole fruit versus fruit juice.

Reading food labels and using food models are effective ways to teach teens about portion sizes and choosing healthier foods. Meal planning and discussing strategies to cope with social events involving food (i.e., lunch, parties, clubs) are helpful. Some patients may have an all-or-nothing attitude toward healthy eating for PCOS and need to be reassured that eating is not perfect; it is acceptable and normal for them to have some high-fat or highly-refined foods once in a while. Keeping food records can also be an effective way for patients to monitor changes in their intake and practice listening to internal cues of appetite regulation. I like to encourage my adolescent patients to "experiment" with their food choices and see what combinations work best for them. Because so many teens already feel overwhelmed with schoolwork, they may be reluctant to use food records. In this case, careful attention to mindful eating including listening to internal cues of hunger and satiety are needed.

When counseling adolescent patients, dietitians will also have to address issues concerning parents. It is very common for parents, not knowing their child has PCOS, to assume their child was heavy because they were eating too much. This results in clients feeling blamed and ashamed about their weight, especially if repeated attempts at weight loss have failed. Often, parents try and regulate their child's intake by telling them when to stop eating and what foods they can or cannot have. I have found this only worsens the self-esteem of teenagers and causes more resentment toward parents. It also results in teens not being able to effectively trust their internal ability to regulate intake. Sometimes teens will admit to sneaking or bingeing on "off-limit" foods to spite parents. Thus food becomes a tactic used to set boundaries and communication with parents. In these situations, referring patients to an individual or family therapist may be needed.

Dietitians will need to set appropriate boundaries with parents to maintain the relationship with the teenage patient. I prefer to have my patients present when addressing parental concerns. That way, patients can trust me knowing that they are not being talked about behind their backs. A goal of treatment is for the teen to assume responsibility for her eating. Parents may need to be educated on the proper diet modifications for PCOS and separate myths from facts. For example, letting a mother know that studies do not show PCOS teens have to eliminate carbohydrates from their diet; that consumption of whole grains actually improves insulin sensitivity. In making dietary changes, teens may gain support from family members who also follow recommended eating plans.

Of course, not all teenagers want to accept responsibility for their eating and are ready to implement changes in their behaviors. In this instance, the use of motivational interviewing is an effective counseling technique dietitians can use to help clients work through ambivalence about behavior change (31). In a non-judgmental and supportive way, dietitians can help patients explore both positive and negative aspects of their behaviors. By using motivational interviewing techniques such as reflective listening, "rolling with resistance," and positive affirmations, dietitians can avoid getting into power struggles with their adolescent patients and guide them toward change through motivation rather than information (31). Other counseling styles such as behavior therapy and cognitive behavior therapy may be used once the adolescent is ready to implement change (31).

PHYSICAL ACTIVITY

Physical activity should be encouraged as it can lower insulin levels and help manage weight. It can also lower stress, prevent chronic disease, and improve body image. In making recommendations for physical activity, the adolescent's struggle with body image and possible resistance to exercise should be kept in mind. For example, some teenagers who are heavy may avoid swimming because they do not want to be seen in public in a bathing suit, and other activities such as running may be to difficult and embarrassing for them to do. Ideally, activities that promote skills that can be maintained throughout life should be encouraged. This may include activities like yoga, pilates, tai chi, karate, tennis, golf, bowling, or walking. In addition, a lot of my adolescent patients find that they move longer and have more fun when listening to music while exercising. Dietitians can emphasize that increasing activity in everyday life is important. For example, pedometers can be used to increase walking or climbing stairs rather than taking elevators. Compliance is best when teens are able to gain support from family members who model physical activity themselves.

In summary, PCOS is a very complicated endocrine disorder that often goes undiagnosed among adolescents. Teenagers with PCOS experience many symptoms that can have a significant and long-term impact on their self-esteem and body image, putting them at a higher risk for the development of an eating disorder. They are also at risk for chronic diseases and infertility later in life, therefore, early recognition and treatment is key. Current diagnostic criteria for PCOS may not be appropriate for adolescents as their symptoms vary at different stages of development and may be seen as a normal part of puberty. Dietitians should be screening *all* their female adolescent patients for PCOS and recommending further diagnostic testing in those they suspect with the syndrome. Once diagnosed, dietitian's need to educate patients on the proper dietary management for PCOS and support them in implementing life-long changes to improve their health and prevent chronic disease.

CHAPTER SUMMARY

- Adolescence is the most vulnerable and influential stage of PCOS.
- Many of the symptoms of PCOS are "normally" experienced during adolescence and can easily be overlooked.
- Current diagnostic criteria for PCOS may not be appropriate for the adolescent population.
- Dietitians should screen all female adolescent patients for PCOS.
- Risk factors include premature pubarche, obesity, ethnicity, and family history.
- Diet and lifestyle changes are the preferred method of treatment of PCOS in adolescence.
- Many factors can influence the eating habits of teenagers with PCOS.
- Dietitian's need to take an empathetic and encouraging approach to counseling adolescent patients.
- The use of metformin has been shown to be an effective method to improve reproductive and metabolic complications of PCOS among adolescents.
- The use of oral contraceptives among young women with PCOS should be prescribed with caution as they can increase triglyceride and total cholesterol levels and possibly increase insulin levels.

REFERENCES

1. Ovalle F, Azziz R. Insulin resistance, polycystic ovary syndrome, and type 2 diabetes mellitus. *Fertil Steril.* 2002;77:1095–1105.
2. Lewy VD, Danadian K, Witchel SF, Arslanian S. Early metabolic abnormalities in adolescent girls with polycystic ovarian syndrome. *J Pediatr.* 2001;138:38–44.
3. Coviello a, Legro R, Dunaif A. Adolescent girls with polycystic ovary syndrome have an increased risk of the metabolic syndrome associated with increasing androgen levels indepent of obesity and insulin resistance. *J Clin Endocrinol Meta. 2006;91:492-497.*

4. Salmi D, Zisser H, Jovanovic L. Screening for and treatment of polycystic ovary syndrome in teenagers. *Exp Biol Med.* 2004;229:469-377.

5. Himelein MJ, Thatcher S. Depression and Body Image among Women with Polycystic Ovary Syndrome. *J Health Psych.* 2006;11(4):613-25.

6. McCluskey S, Evans C, Lacey JH, Pearce JM, Jacobs H. Polycystic ovary syndrome and bulimia. *Fertil Steril.* 1991;55:287–291.

7. Warren-Ulanch J, Arslanian S. Treatment of PCOS in adolescence. *Best practice and Research Clinical Endocrinology and Metabolism.* 2006;20(2):311-330.

8. The Rotterdam ESHRE/ASRM sponsored PCOS consensus workshop group: revised 2003 consensus on diagnostic criteria and long term health risks related to polycystic ovary syndrome. *Fertil Steril.* 2004;81:19-25.

9. Driscoll D. Polycystic ovary syndrome in adolescence. *Seminars in reproductive medicine.* 2003;21(3):301-307.

10. Katherine D. Sherif, M.D.Ppersonal communication, September 2006.

11. Lego RS, Finegood D, Dunaif A. A fasting glucose to insulin ratio is a useful measure of insulin sensitivity in women with polycystic ovary syndrome. *J Clin Endocrinol Metab.* 1998;83:2694-2698.

12. Pfeifer S. Polycystic ovary syndrome in adolescent girls. *Seminars in Ped Surgery.* 2005;14:111-117.

13. Apter D, Vihko R. Premenarcheal endocrine changes in relation to age at menarche. *Clinical Endocrinol (Oxford).* 1985;22:753-760.

14. Dieudonne MN, Pecquery R, Boumediene A, Leneveu MC. Androgen receptors in human preadipocytes and adipocytes: regional specificities and regulation by sex steroids. *Am J Physiol.* 1998;274:C1645-C1652.

15. Kent SC, Legro RS. Polycystic ovary syndrome in adolescents. *Adolesc Med.* 2002;13:73–88.

16. Ibáñez L, Valls C, Marcos MV, Ong K, Dunger D, Zegher F. Insulin sensitization for girls with precocious pubarche and with risk for polycystic ovary syndrome: effects of prepubertal initiation and post-pubertal discontinuation of metformin treatment . *J of Clin Endocrinol Metab.* 2004;89(9): 4331-4337.

17. Kashar-Miller MD, Nixon C, Boots LR, Go RC, Azzia R. Prevalence of

polycystic ovary syndrome (PCOS) in first-degree relatives of patients with PCOS. *Fertil Steril.* 2001;75:53-58.

18. Meo R, Bilo L. Polycystic ovary syndrome and epilepsy: a review of the evidence. *Drugs.* 2003;63:1185–1227.

19. Kolodziejezyk, B et al, Metformin therapy decreases hyperandrogenism and hyperinsulinemia in women with polycystic ovary syndrome. *Fertil Steril. 2002;* 73(6):1149-54.

20. De Leo V, Musacchio MC, Morgante G, Piomboni P, Petraglia F. Metformin treatment is effective in obese teenage girls with PCOS. *Hum Reprod.* 2006;185(1).

21. Arslanian SA, Lewy V, Danadian K, Saad R. Metformin therapy in obese adolescents with polycystic ovary syndrome and impaired glucose tolerance: amelioration of exaggerated adrenal response to adrenocorticotropin with reduction of insulinemia/insulin resistance. *J Clin Endocrinol Metab.* 2002;87:1555–1559.

22. Glueck CJ, Wang P, Fontaine R, Tracy T, Sieve-Smith L. Merformin to restore normal menses in oligoamenorrheic teenage girls with polycystic ovary syndrome (PCOS). *J Adolesc Health.* 2001;29:160–169.

23. Romualdi D, Guido M, Ciampelli M, Giuliani M, Leoni F, Perri C, Lanzone A. Selective effects of pioglitazone on insulin and androgen abnormalities in normo- and hyperinsulinaemic obese patients with polycystic ovary syndrome. *Hum Reprod.* 2003;18:1210–1218.

24. Glueck CJ, Moreira A, Goldenberg N, Sieve L, Wang P. Pioglitazone and metformin in obese women with polycystic ovary syndrome not optimally responsive to metformin. *Hum Reprod.* 2003;18:1618–1625.

25. Food and Drug Administration. FDA Issues Safety Alert on Avandia. www.fda.gov. Accessed May, 21, 2007.

26. Jensen JT, Speroff L. Health benefits of oral contraceptives. *Obstet Gynecol Clin North Am.* 2000;27:705–721.

27. Cagnacci A, Paoletti AM, Renzi A, Orru M, Pilloni M, Meilis GB, Volpe A. Glucose metabolism and insulin resistance in women with polycystic ovary syndrome during therapy with oral contraceptives containing cyproterone acetate or desogesterel. *J of Clin Endocrinol Metab.* 2005;88(8):3621-3625.

28. Marsh K, Brand-Miller J. The optimal diet for women with polycystic ovary syndrome. *British J of Nutrition.* 2005;94:154-165.

29. Omichinski L. Polycystic Ovary Syndrome: An Open Door for

Dietetics Professionals (seminar). Food and Nutrition Conference, Denver, CO 2000.

30. Spears BA. Does Dieting Increase the Risk for Obesity and Eating Disorders?
    *J Amer Diet Assoc.*2006;106(4):523-525.

31. Resnicow K, Davis R, Rollnick S. Motivational interviewing for pediatric obesity: conceptual issues and evidence review. *J Am Diet Assoc.* 2006;106:2024-2033.

32. Jahanfar S, et al. Bulimia Nervosa and Polycystic Ovary Syndrome. *Gynecol. Endocrinol.* 1995;9:113-117.

CHAPTER 7

PREGNANCY, LACTATION, AND THE POSTPARTUM PERIOD

THERE ARE MANY FACTORS to take into consideration when a woman with PCOS becomes pregnant. This is a very exciting time for these women, especially because so many of them may have been trying to conceive with or without fertility treatments for years. In addition, becoming pregnant is a definite sign of femininity and it may be a relief to some women who have been feeling very masculine over the years due to their "male" shape and their symptoms of excess hair growth and balding. Having PCOS and being pregnant, however, may pose some risks. Some women who have undergone fertility treatments may be carrying multiple babies and will have special dietary and medical concerns. Also, because many women with PCOS have hormonal imbalances and are overweight or obese, they are at a higher risk for miscarriage (1-3) and complications such as gestational diabetes (GDM) and hypertensive disorders during pregnancy (4-6). Proper medical management and medical nutrition therapy (MNT) are imperative to prevent the onset of these complications and to optimize fetal growth and development. This chapter discusses the nutritional and medical concerns women with PCOS may face during pregnancy and lactation. Suggested dietary guidelines for these women are provided. Weight management during the postpartum period is also discussed.

POLYCYSTIC OVARY SYNDROME AND PREGNANCY

EMOTIONAL CONCERNS IN PREGNANCY

Many women with PCOS who are able to conceive may have many misconceptions when it comes to a healthy diet during pregnancy. Although current evidence does not support it, popular diet guidelines for PCOS (mostly from the internet) recommend a very low-carbohydrate diet. This may be problematic for some women who followed these recommendations, as they may feel apprehensive about eating foods containing carbohydrates during pregnancy. This includes fruits, vegetables, legumes, and grains, all of which provide important vitamins, minerals, and fiber and are essential for fetal growth and development. Pregnancy is not the time to be fearful of carbohydrates. Women may also be inclined to limit carbohydrates out of fear of gaining too much weight or to prevent the onset of gestational diabetes (currently no evidence supports the notion of limiting carbohydrates during pregnancy to prevent gestational diabetes). For these reasons, dietitians should screen patients with PCOS for negative attitudes toward food and weight, conveying the importance of consuming whole grain carbohydrates in sufficient amounts.

Some women, on the other hand, might find pregnancy a license to eat anything they want as they may, for the first time ever, feel less pressure to restrict their intake in a society obsessed with thinness. This can be troublesome if they have been very restrictive in their eating prior to conceiving. It can lead to bingeing during pregnancy, resulting in excessive weight gain. Additionally, women who already struggle with anxiety and depression may feel these conditions are exasperated during pregnancy and could turn to food for emotional support. A recent study published in the *Journal of the American Dietetic Association* found that pregnant women who reported high stress, anxiety, and fatigue consumed more carbohydrates, fats, and protein and less vitamin C and folate (7). It is common for a woman who has been following a diet of limited or primarily whole grain carbohydrates pre-pregnancy to abandon this way of eating while pregnant, turning to refined carbohydrates and saturated fat-containing foods because, as one patient put it, "I am pregnant now and do not have to worry about managing my insulin levels or watching what I eat." This attitude is problematic as it can lead to excessive weight gain during pregnancy, increasing the chances of adverse health risks.

Body image issues can also be a concern during pregnancy as those who have struggled with their weight most of their lives may feel that the weight gain will get out of control. They may also have difficulties accepting weight gain and getting larger in general. Proper education of "where the weight goes" during pregnancy (see Table 1), can be very helpful to reassure clients that weight gain is necessary and healthy if gained in reasonable amounts. These women also carry their weight in their mid-section and may not look pregnant until their third trimester causing some to struggle with body image issues of failing to look pregnant. One PCOS patient I worked with who was pregnant admitted to purposely wanting to eat extra food to gain more weight than she already had because she wasn't "showing" yet, and wanted the attention she saw other pregnant women receive. This patient was in the middle of her second trimester and had gained a reasonable seven pounds.

In addition to normal emotional variations due to fluctuating hormone levels, pregnancy is full of different emotions for the PCOS woman. Dietitians and other health professionals need to screen PCOS women for possible eating and body image issues to ensure proper fetal growth and development. Patients can benefit from working with a dietitian to understand reasonable weight gain goals, body changes, and proper diet for a healthy pregnancy.

Table 1. Distribution of total weight gain during pregnancy			
Mother		Fetus	
Uterus	2 lb	Baby	7.5-8.5 lb
Breasts	1 lb	Placenta	1.5 lb
Blood	4 lb	Amniotic fluid	2.0 lb
Tissue fluids	3 lb		
Fat stores	7 lb		

Reference 8

HEALTH CONCERNS OF PREGNANT WOMEN WITH POLYCYSTIC OVARY SYNDROME

The National Institutes of Health (NIH) defines PCOS as a state of hyperandrogenic chronic anovulation, leading some obstetricians to believe that PCOS does not really exist once a woman becomes pregnant (certainly, they must have ovulated to become pregnant) (9). Thus, they may not consider a pregnant woman with PCOS a high-risk pregnancy. Although the exact mechanisms have not been identified, it has long been established that women who are overweight or obese are at a higher risk of complications during pregnancy including gestational diabetes (GDM) (10), congenital malformations (11), prolonged labor (12), cesarean sections (13-15), macrosomia (infant born weighing > 4000 grams) (16), pregnancy induced hypertension (PIH), and pre-eclampsia (3). Many have questioned whether women with PCOS, who typically are overweight or obese and have hyperinsulinanemia and insulin resistance, are at a higher risk for developing adverse outcomes during pregnancy. So far only a limited number of studies have been conducted to determine this and the results are conflicting (17-20). The most recent study involved a group of 66 pregnant women with PCOS and age and weight matched controls (17). No significant differences were found among complications of GDM, PIH, and premature deliveries between the PCOS pregnant women and controls (17). In contrast, the largest study involving 99 PCOS pregnancies found no differences in the rate of pre-eclampsia but a slightly increased risk GDM (19). In most of the studies, the most important risk factor for GDM was body mass index (BMI).

GESTATIONAL DIABETES AND POLYCYSTIC OVARY SYNDROME

Gestational diabetes is defined as any degree of glucose intolerance with onset or first recognition during pregnancy (21). GDM exists in approximately 7% of all pregnancies (22). It is associated with increased risk of fetal macrosomia, increasing the need for cesarean births and the risk of maternal hypertensive disorders (22). Long-term risks of having GDM include maternal development of type 2 diabetes (T2DM), and in babies born to mothers with GDM, an increased risk of obesity, glucose intolerance, and diabetes in late adolescence (22).

As discussed earlier, despite conflicting research suggesting women with PCOS have higher incidences of GDM, higher rates of hyperinsulinemia and insulin resistance do exist among the PCOS population. Because of this, many physicians I have worked with usually recommended that an oral glucose tolerance test (OGTT) be initiated earlier in PCOS women. They recommend testing at 20 weeks gestation to screen for GDM and, if normal, be repeated by the standard screening time for all pregnant women, between 24-28 weeks gestation. The diagnostic criteria for GDM with either a 75-gram or 100-gram oral glucose load is shown in Tables 2 and 3. Some practitioners may even require a glucose screen earlier, at the initial visit. According to the American Diabetes Association, a fasting plasma glucose level > 126 mg/dl or a casual plasma glucose > 200 mg/dl meets the diagnosis criteria for diabetes and requires no further glucose testing (22). Also, it is advisable for these women to continue or begin taking metformin throughout their pregnancies as a preventative measure to control insulin levels and possibly avoid GDM (23). Metformin has been shown to be safe in patients with PCOS throughout pregnancy. Lactic acidosis is a rare side effect, occurring in .03 cases per 1,000 patient-years (23).

Table 2. Diagnosis of gestational diabetes mellitus with a 100-gram oral glucose load

Time	Plasma Glucose Goals (mg/dl)
Fasting	95
1-h	180
2-h	155
3h	140

Two or more of the venous plasma concentrations must be met or exceeded for a positive diagnosis. The test should be done in the morning after an overnight fast of between 8 and 14 h and after at least 3 days of unrestricted diet ($\geq$150 g carbohydrate per day) and unlimited physical activity. The subject should remain seated and should not smoke throughout the test. Reprinted from The American Diabetes Association: Gestational diabetes mellitus [Position statement], *Diabetes Care.* 2004;27:S88-90.

Table 3. Diagnosis of gestational diabetes mellitus with a 75-g oral glucose load

Time	Plasma Glucose Goals (mg/dl)
Fasting	95
1-h	180
2-h	155

Two or more of the venous plasma concentrations must be met or exceeded for a positive diagnosis. The test should be done in the morning after an overnight fast of between 8 and 14 h and after at least 3 days of unrestricted diet ($\geq$ 150 g carbohydrate per day) and unlimited physical activity. The subject should remain seated and should not smoke throughout the test. Reprinted from The American Diabetes Association: Gestational diabetes mellitus [Position statement], *Diabetes Care.* 2004;27:S88-90.

All women with GDM should receive nutritional counseling from a registered dietitian on an appropriate diet that provides adequate calories and nutrients for the demands of pregnancy and that are consistent with established blood glucose goals (22). Urinary ketone monitoring can indicate whether the patient is consuming sufficient calories or carbohydrates if they are following a calorie restricted diet (22). Exercise of any form can help with insulin resistance and controlling postprandial hyperglycemia, especially if done after eating. One example is walking after meals for 10-20 minutes. If glucose levels do not improve with diet and exercise, the use of human insulin may be needed. The American Diabetes Association does not currently recommend the use of oral glucose-lowering agents during pregnancy in patients with GDM or type 2 diabetes (T2DM) (22,23). However, many physicians have been recommending the use of metformin during pregnancy with their PCOS patients to reduce the risk of miscarriage and GDM (23).

WEIGHT GAIN RECOMMENDATIONS FOR WOMEN WITH POLYCYSTIC OVARY SYNDROME

There is a significant amount of literature demonstrating the association between increased complications during pregnancy due to obesity, yet little attention has been shown to the management of weight gain during and after pregnancy. In 1990, the Institute of Medicine (IOM) came out with weight gain recommendations based on BMI advising women with a "normal" BMI of 19.8-26.0 kg/m2 to gain approximately 25-35 lbs (about one pound per week) throughout their entire pregnancy (24). Those considered over-weight with a BMI of 26.1-29.0 kg/m2 are advised to gain 15-25 lbs and those with a BMI > 29 kg/m2 (obese) should gain approximately 15 lbs during the course of pregnancy. Women considered under-weight (BMI < 19.8 kg/m2) are to gain 28-40 lbs (24) (see Table 4). Some researchers have criticized these guidelines, implying that they are too generous and fail to consider the potential adverse effects of excessive weight gain during pregnancy and do not provide specific recommendations for women with extreme obesity (BMI $\geq$ 40 kg/m2) (25,26). Additionally, there are no formal recommendations available regarding weight gain for overweight or obese women pregnant with multiples, which is common among PCOS women as they often undergo fertility treatments to conceive.

Table 4. Weight gain recommendations during pregnancy by weight status

Weight Status	Total Weight Gain
Underweight (BMI < 19.8 kg/m2)	28-40 lbs
Normal weight (BMI 19.8 to 26 kg/m2)	25-35 lbs
Overweight (BMI 26 kg/m2 to 29 kg/m2)	15-25 lbs
Obese (BMI > 29 kg/m2)	15 lbs
Twin gestation	35-45 lbs
Triplet gestation	45-55 lbs

Reference 24

Since the release of the IOM guidelines, it has been documented that the majority of women exceed these recommendations (27,28). One study showed that 57% of white, 61% of black, and 51% of Latina pregnant women exceeded the IOM weight gain recommendations (29). Excessive prenatal weight gain increases the risk for postpartum weight retention and obstetrical complications such as macrosomia, which can lead to shoulder dystocia and increases the need for cesarean section (30).

As shown in Table 1, the average amount of fat stores women gain in preparation for pregnancy and lactation is 7 pounds with most of that weight gained between 10 and 20 weeks gestation (8). Most of the excess weight women gain in pregnancy is related to an increase in fat stores (31). The more fat stores a woman has, the longer it could take her to lose the weight postpartum and return to her pre-pregnancy weight (28). Because many women with PCOS are overweight, they already have the necessary fat stores in place for pregnancy and may not need to gain weight until later in their second or even third trimester. Even then, it is possible for some obese women to gain hardly any weight throughout the entire pregnancy and still deliver healthy full-term babies (9). I have found that regular exercise and carefully following a diet that limits calories but still provides enough energy for optimal fetal growth and development can help patients achieve this, along with close monitoring of the development of the fetus. It is important to note that low weight gain in the second or third trimester increases the risk for intrauterine growth retardation and preterm delivery (32). Therefore, maternal weight gain recommendations should be individualized according to the physician, taking into consideration the client's pre-pregnancy BMI, age, race, activity level, rate of weight gain, and any potential risk of adverse complications in pregnancy.

MEDICAL NUTRITION THERAPY FOR POLYCYSTIC OVARY SYNDROME IN PREGNANCY

THE DIET PLAN

Currently, there are no formal MNT recommendations for PCOS during pregnancy. In general, the nutrition guidelines I have been recommending to women with PCOS during pregnancy are similar to that of the diet guidelines for someone who has PCOS when not pregnant. These recommendations resemble the dietary treatment of gestational diabetes, which emphasize:

- Eating a variety of foods
- Whole grain and high fiber foods including breads, cereals, fruits, legumes, and vegetables spread evenly throughout the day
- Limited intake of simple sugars including sweets and sweetened beverages (soda, juices, juice drinks, sports drinks)
- Eating often, every 3-5 hours spread out between 3 small meals and 2 to 4 snacks
- Consuming protein with all meals and snacks
- 600 mcg of folic acid daily
- 1000 mg of calcium daily
- Adequate intakes of essential fatty acids (including omega-3s)
- Adequate fluids
- Limited caffeine intake (<300 mg/day)
- Avoidance of alcohol, smoking, and illegal drugs
- Limited intake of artificial sweeteners
- Limited intake of seafood containing methylmercury (tuna, shark, swordfish, tilefish)
- Avoidance of unpasteurized juices and milk products, including soft cheeses

CALORIC REQUIREMENTS FOR PREGNANT WOMEN WITH POLYCYSTIC OVARY SYNDROME

The phrase "eating for two" is a widespread myth. While an adequate dietary intake for pregnant women is critical for optimal fetal growth and development, eating excessive amounts of calories is not ideal. For most women, energy needs during pregnancy range between 2,500 to 2,700 calories a day, but like weight gain recommendations, other factors must be considered including pre-pregnancy BMI, rate of weight gain, maternal age, and appetite (33). It is very important for dietitians to work collaboratively with PCOS patients to prevent excessive weight gain during pregnancy especially if the patient is overweight or obese prior to conception. Many women who become pregnant may be unaware of the adverse effects of excess weight gain to them or their babies.

Currently, there are limited dietary recommendations for American women who are obese during pregnancy. The American Dietetic Association recommends that obese women (BMI > 29) consume approximately 25 kcal/kg actual body weight (33). Overweight or obese women pregnant with multiples are to consult with their physician for specific caloric intakes and weight gain recommendations. The NIH and the U.S. Department of Health and Human Services have provided dietary guidelines for pregnancy suggesting that women not increase their daily caloric intake in the first 3 months of pregnancy (34).Women who were at a normal weight prior to conception are to increase their intake an average of 300 calories in the 2nd and 3rd trimesters. According to The American Dietetic Association, however, some normal and overweight women may need less than the extra 300 calories a day, especially those that are sedentary (33), further supporting the need for moderate weight gain in pregnancy. They suggest relying on appetite instead as a better indicator of energy sufficiency (33).

Therefore, dietetic professionals should encourage their pregnant patients to recognize and trust their own hunger and satiety cues to determine how much food they need. This can be done by having clients rate and record their level of hunger and satiety before and after meals according to a number scale. For example, a scale of zero to 10 where zero is completely starving and 10 meaning Thanksgiving dinner stuffed. The idea is for patients to recognize when they need food and respond to this need in a timely matter, not waiting so long that they are extremely hungry which only results in greater food consumption. It also helps patients to recognize when they do not need any more food and to stop eating, which can prevent episodes of binge eating. In addition, it may be helpful for dietetics practitioners to demonstrate conscious eating in nutrition sessions with their patients for them to practice at home. More information on this can be found in Chapter 8.

Unfortunately, conscious eating can be difficult for PCOS patients who have spent years of their lives dieting and trusting the rules of a diet to determine when, what and how much they are allowed to eat. This can result in them not being able to recognize when they are starting to get hungry or whether they are full, leading to excessive calorie consumption. In these situations, patients may benefit from more structure in the form of a meal plan that explains appropriate ranges of food exchanges while listening to internal cues of hunger and satiety as the ultimate guide to determining food intake. Meeting regularly with a dietitian who can assess food logs, discuss conscious eating, and explore feelings associated with specific meals, can provide support to PCOS patients in achieving appropriate weight gain in pregnancy.

CARBOHYDRATE REQUIREMENTS FOR PREGNANCY

Because it has been shown to reduce maternal glucose levels and improve maternal and fetal outcomes (34,35), it is generally recommended that women with GDM and obese women with or without GDM not only reduce their calories during pregnancy, but also reduce carbohydrate intake to 35-40% of total calories (33). This would mean that a pregnant woman who is 5'5" and weighs 247 lbs. (112 kg) would need up to 2,800 calories per day (using 25 kcal/kg actual body weight), and between 245 and 280 grams of carbohydrates per day. Consuming too few carbohydrates is not advisable, as they provide energy and fiber as well as essential vitamins and minerals (grains, for example, are main sources of folate). Most importantly, maternal glucose is the primary energy source for intrauterine growth (36). The Estimated Average Requirement (EAR) for carbohydrates is 135 grams/day (36), to meet the demands of the fetus' brain, prevent ketosis, and maintain appropriate blood glucose levels (38). One study found that women who consumed too few amounts of a lower glycemic index (GI) diet had reduced infant birth weight (39).

The type of carbohydrate consumed during pregnancy is of utmost importance. A recent study published in the *American Journal of Clinical Nutrition* indicated that a low GI diet may favorably influence long-term outcomes in babies (36). Seventy healthy pregnant women between 12 and 16 weeks gestation with a single fetus were assigned to either a moderately high or low GI diet. Those following the high GI diet delivered infants who were heavier and more likely to be large-for-gestational age (3% versus 33%). Additionally, although within normal levels for both groups, serum glucose was found to be lower among the women in the low GI group (36). There was no effect of diet composition on maternal weight gain, method of delivery or measures of insulin sensitivity (36). The researchers suggest that since babies who are born large-for-gestational age are at a higher risk for developing obesity and chronic diseases later in life, consuming a low GI diet during pregnancy would be beneficial to improve fetal outcomes (36).

A low GI diet can not only improve fetal outcomes, but may even reduce the risk of the mother developing GDM (40). A prospective cohort study involving 13,110 women from the Nurses' Health Study II showed a 26% reduction in GDM risk for every 10 gram per day increment in dietary fiber (40). The authors suggest that fiber has a beneficial effect on glucose homeostasis by possibly delaying gastric emptying which slows glucose absorption, thus lessening the need for more insulin (40). Normally, a state of insulin resistance develops in the third trimester of pregnancy as higher levels of glucose are utilized to meet fetal demands. This study also found that each 5 gram/day increment in fruit fiber was associated with a 26% reduction in risk for GDM (40).

Like the treatment for GDM, it is important for dietetic professionals to convey to their pregnant PCOS patients the importance of distributing carbohydrates evenly throughout the day. Typically, this is represented by three meals and between two and four snacks, with the inclusion of an evening snack to manage glucose levels through the night. All meals and snacks need to include protein-rich foods to help stabilize glucose levels. Because of the high rate of miscarriage in PCOS related to elevated insulin levels, simple carbohydrates, including sweetened beverages (juices, soft drinks, sports drinks), candies, and desserts should be limited and avoided when possible. Since very limited data exists regarding PCOS and pregnancy, dietary recommendations must be drawn from other studies involving the effects of carbohydrates on insulin and glucose levels in pregnancy. I recommend my PCOS patients who are pregnant consume a carbohydrate intake of 35-40% of total calories, based on the related evidence discussed and consistent with The American Diabetes Association guidelines for GDM (33). The majority of carbohydrates should be of high fiber quality, with at least 28 grams each day (the DRI requirement) for optimal glucose and insulin control.

PROTEIN NEEDS FOR PREGNANCY

The RDA for protein during pregnancy is 1.1 grams per kilogram of body weight or 71 grams per day (37). Good sources of protein include meat, poultry, seafood, soy, nuts and legumes which also provide good sources of iron, zinc and magnesium. Those that are lactose intolerant can choose dairy foods containing less lactose such as cheese, yogurt, soy milk or milk with added lactase enzyme (33). Women who are pregnant and nursing mothers should avoid shark, swordfish, king mackerel, and tilefish (also called golden bass), which may contain high levels of methylmercury. Mercury, which is passed to the fetus through a mothers' blood, is toxic to fetal brain development. Women should also limit consumption of other fatty fish to 12 ounces per week or about 3-4 servings/week.

ESSENTIAL FATTY ACIDS FOR PREGNANCY

Consuming adequate amounts of essential fatty acids during pregnancy is imperative for all mothers as they play an important role in infant reproductive, brain, and visual functions and may reduce the incidence of PIH (42). Currently, the DRI for linoleic acid (omega-6 fatty acids) is 13 grams and 1.4 grams for alpha-linolenic acid (omega-3 fatty acids) during pregnancy (37). It has been established that most Americans consume sufficient amounts of omega-6 fatty acids in their diets yet lack adequate amounts of omega-3 fatty acids. An ideal ratio of omega-3 fatty acids to omega-6 is 3:1. Vegetarian women do not usually have adequate sources of omega-3 fatty acids since their diets do not contain fish. In fact, lower levels of docosahexaenoic acid (DHA) have been reported in infants born to vegetarian mothers (41).

Good sources of omega-3 fatty acids that are safe for women to eat during pregnancy include freshly ground flax seed and unprocessed flax seed oil, walnuts, butternuts, cold-pressed, unrefined canola and soybean oils as well as salmon (limited to 12 ounces per week). Other sources include cod liver oil, egg yolks and organ meats. Many prenatal vitamins now include omega-6 and omega-3 fatty acids.

It has been established that DHA is important in vision development, especially in the last trimester of pregnancy. Vision has found to be impaired in infants born prematurely who lack adequate amounts of DHA in the retina (43). Research now shows that both omega-6 and omega-3 fatty acids decrease significantly during pregnancy as women have difficulty keeping up with the high demand, especially for DHA (42). It also appears that the more fetuses a women carries, the more depleted she is of essential fatty acids. Once stores are compromised, they are slow to recover unless extra DHA supplementation is given (42). For these reasons, it is recommended that pregnant women consume not only a diet consisting of sufficient essential fatty acids to meet her needs, but that of her fetus as well (42,43). In addition, it may be beneficial for women to continue supplementing their diets with omega-3 and 6 fatty acids for the first 6 months after giving birth (42). Future research is needed to determine optimal dosage amounts (42).

THE USE OF ALTERNATIVE REMEDIES IN PREGNANCY

It is popular among women with PCOS to take herbal and botanical products to treat symptoms and possibly increase fertility. Some women may wish to continue taking them during pregnancy, especially if they deem them safe or natural. Those who were able to conceive while taking alternative treatments may want to continue taking them in hopes that they will help support a healthy pregnancy. As mentioned in Chapter 5, however, the safety and effectiveness of the majority of these products have not been documented or studied in pregnant and lactating women and should be viewed as drugs. Manufacturers do not currently have to prove their safety for use among pregnant or nursing women. Many of these herbs like black cohosh, chasteberry, and fenugreek can alter hormone levels and stimulate uterine contractions. A list of some common herbs and botanicals that are contraindicated in pregnancy are listed in Table 5. Many of these products are used among the PCOS community. The American Academy of Pediatrics also recommends that pregnant women limit the consumption of herbal teas to two 8-oz. servings per day, and advise pregnant women to choose herbal teas in filtered tea bags (44).

Table 5. Some herbal and botanical supplements to avoid during pregnancy

Agnus castus	Ginseng
Cayenne pepper	Feverfew
Chamomile	Hawthorne
Black cohosh	Licorice
Blue cohosh	Motherwort
Comfrey	Red clover
Dong quai	Sassafras
Echinacea	St. John's wort
Fenugreek	Valerian root
Fennel	Vervain

References: 45,46

EXERCISE IN PREGNANCY

It is currently recommended that pregnant women engage in at least 30 minutes of moderate physical activity on most days of the week (47). Pregnant PCOS women can reap the benefits of physical exercise including weight management, increased physical fitness (sure to help with the demands of labor and recovery), reduced risk of developing GDM and PIH, as well as psychological well-being (33). In addition, moderate physical activity during pregnancy has been shown to lower maternal glucose levels in women with GDM (22). Women who have not been exercising prior to pregnancy should consult with their doctors before starting an exercise program.

Low to moderately intense activities that are safe for pregnant women include walking, running, swimming, tennis, biking, yoga, and pilates. Activities that could cause abdominal trauma or falling are contraindicated in pregnancy and include skiing, martial arts, scuba diving, and any exercise over 2,500 meters of altitude. Women with PIH, toxemia, pre-eclampsia, preterm rupture of membranes, history of preterm labor, second or third trimester persistant bleeding, incompetent cervix, or any intrauterine growth retardation should not exercise (33). Pregnant women who exercise need to maintain adequate caloric and fluid needs and maintain a heart rate at 60% to 80% of maximum (220 minus age = maximum heart rate) (33).

METFORMIN AND PREGNANCY

Many women with PCOS take metformin (glucophage®, Bristol-Myers Squibb Co.) to help reduce their insulin levels before getting pregnant and it is very common for these women to conceive while on the medication as well. Metformin has been shown to be beneficial in increasing ovulation rates in women with PCOS with or without clomid as it can reduce insulin levels causing androgen levels to be suppressed at the ovaries (23). Until recently, it was advisable for women taking metformin to discontinue its use during pregnancy. Diabetics who were taking metformin were advised to discontinue it, and use insulin instead to manage their blood sugars during pregnancy. This was because of fears of potential fetal teratogenicity and possible hypoglycemic effects on the fetus from taking a hypoglycemic agent (23). Thanks to significant research, metformin is not only safe for women with PCOS to take during pregnancy and even beneficial to both mother and fetus. It is certainly a more convenient alternative than insulin (23).

Metformin is a biguanide and reduces serum glucose by reducing the production of glucose at the liver by inhibiting gluconeogenesis and reducing peripheral insulin resistance (48). Metformin has not been shown to cause hypoglycemia because it does not enhance endogenous insulin production (23). It also does not appear to stimulate fetal beta pancreatic cells to produce insulin or cause hypoglycemia in fetuses or in newborns (49). No evidence of adverse neonatal affects or teratogenicity have been associated with metformin use among women with PCOS (1). At dosages between 1.5-2.55 g/day, metformin has not been shown to affect newborns' birth weight, length, growth, or motor-social development when 126 infants the first 18 months of life were compared to the normal U.S. infant population (50).

Women with PCOS are at a 30-50% increased risk of miscarriage (before 12 weeks gestation) in addition to low conception rates due mostly to elevated insulin levels (1-3). Current studies demonstrate a significant reduction in the incidence of first-trimester miscarriages in PCOS women who were taking metformin during conception and throughout pregnancy. In one study involving PCOS pregnant women and metformin, 65 pregnant PCOS women were placed in a metformin-treated group and 35 were the control group with no metformin. All subjects were matched for age, BMI, serum insulin and testosterone levels. The rate of first-trimester miscarriages was significantly reduced in the metformin-treated group compared to the control group (8.8% vs. 42.9%) (1). The researchers suggest metformin is beneficial in preventing miscarriage in women with PCOS by reducing insulin levels.

Other benefits of its use during pregnancy is that metformin has been shown to reduce the incidence of pre-eclampsia, macrosomia, and the chances of PCOS women developing GDM (23,50). In a study of 95 live births, the development of GDM in women with PCOS who took metformin during pregnancy was lower than that of controls (9.5% vs. 15.9%) (50). The researchers suggest that meformin helps to prevent GDM and improve pregnancy outcomes in women with PCOS by helping to reduce pre-conception and pregnancy weight gain, insulin resistance and secretion, by reducing hyperinsulinanemia (50).

POLYCYSTIC OVARY SYNDROME AND LACTATION

DO WOMEN WITH PCOS HAVE MORE DIFFICULTY BREAST FEEDING?

Because of the many hormonal imbalances associated with PCOS, it has been speculated that some women with the syndrome may have difficulty breastfeeding and producing an adequate milk supply for their infants. The hormonal aberrations in PCOS involve insulin, progesterone, and estrogen, all of which are also important to breast development and milk secreting ability (51). Lisa Marasco, MA, IBCLC, is a lactation consultant who began studying the connection between PCOS and low milk supply after seeing two PCOS patients within one day who had problems with low milk production. In her thesis, she studied a group of 30 women with lactation failure and found that over half of them were obese, 57% had a history of infertility, and 67% experienced oligo- or amenorrhea (51). According to Marasco, some women with PCOS may have more difficulties producing adequate milk because the breast tissue fails to undergo the normal physiological changes during pregnancy needed to prepare for lactation, or perhaps not enough breast tissue existed prior to pregnancy (52). It is known that women with PCOS have low levels of progesterone which is needed for alveolar growth and development in breast tissue. Insulin also plays a role in milk production and having insulin resistance may also contribute to lactation problems in women with PCOS (51).

Lactation consultants recommend that all women with PCOS pump after feedings for at least 10-15 minutes on each breast to help establish an adequate milk supply in the first 2 weeks of initiating nursing. This is due to the potential difficulties women with PCOS may face with breastfeeding and because nursing is encouraged for its numerous benefits to mother and infant. Frequent feedings with full drainage can also help maximize milk production as well as drinking at least 16 eight-ounce glasses of water (16 ounces at each nursing session) each day and eating an adequate diet. One study showed that the volume of milk production is decreased when caloric intake drops below 1500 calories per day (54). For mothers with a low milk supply, extra breast stimulation by frequent nursing or pumping sessions is crucial.

Milk supply problems may be prevented or ameliorated by establishing early intervention strategies during pregnancy. This may include obtaining resources for local breastfeeding support groups, and preparing to work with a board-certified lactation consultant soon after giving birth. Good breastfeeding management including proper latch and positioning are imperative to successful milk production and proper infant growth and development.

According to Marasco, all of these tactics will help establish the foundation to good milk supply, yet they do not address the underlying problems (52). Although not scientifically tested, goat's rue, fennel, kale, verbena, chasteberry, and fenugreek (see Chapter 5) are herbal supplements reputed to increase milk supply and possibly stimulate breast growth (53,55). The use of progesterone supplements and metformin during pregnancy have also been speculated to help support an adequate milk supply in PCOS women and possibly support breast development during pregnancy, but also has not yet been proven (51). Marasco claims she has tried metformin with "a number of PCOS moms with low supply, and in some cases metformin alone increases milk production (52)." But she adds, "metformin is not going to help much if the woman does not have enough breast tissue in place to begin with (52)." Medications such as Reglan® (metoclopramide) can also be prescribed to boost the milk supply (52,53). Interestingly, as some women with PCOS experience low milk supply, others are reporting an overabundance of milk production. Obviously, this is an area that needs much more research.

IS METFORMIN SAFE TO USE WHILE BREAST FEEDING?

Since many women choose to take metformin during pregnancy for the many health benefits discussed earlier, they may be inclined to continue taking metformin while they breastfeed to prevent "rebounding" of PCOS symptoms after birth, control insulin levels, and possibly help to produce an adequate milk supply. However, the use of metformin during lactation is still controversial.

Not surprisingly, limited information exists about whether metformin is safe to take while breastfeeding as the risks to the infant are still unknown. The few studies that are available have consisted of relatively limited sample sizes and results show that metformin does cross into the milk supply but in amounts that appear to be "clinically insignificant" with no adverse affects to infants (55-58). The most recent and largest study was conducted among 61 nursing infants and 50 formula fed infants born to mothers with PCOS who took an average of 2.55 grams of metformin per day throughout pregnancy and lactation (59). The infants were followed up to 6 months of age with results showing that the breastfed infants of mothers who took metformin had no adverse health risks in regards to growth or motor-social development (59).

In researching this book, however, the numerous pediatricians, obstetricians, and reproductive endocrinologists I have interviewed have offered conflicting advice on whether to take metformin while nursing. Some physicians do not feel comfortable advising women to breastfeed while taking the medication because of the lack of evidence supporting the safety of metformin while breastfeeding, especially because it has been documented that metformin does cross into the milk supply. Other physicians say they have been instructing mom's to breastfeed on metformin as infants have already been exposed to it in utero because metformin does cross the placenta, and because it does not appear to be teratogenic, cause hypoglycemia or any adverse health risks. Basically, until more long-term and larger studies are conducted, women with PCOS who do plan to breastfeed while on metformin should discuss their options with their physician and care-fully make a risk-benefit analysis before beginning breastfeeding. If a woman does decide to take metformin while nursing, frequent monitoring of the infants health and feeding habits are advisable (57,58).

POSTPARTUM WEIGHT MANAGEMENT FOR MOTHERS WITH POLYCYSTIC OVARY SYNDROME

Studies suggest that the greater amount of weight a women gains during her pregnancy, the more likely she is to retain the weight postpartum (60,61). Being at a higher weight between pregnancies may contribute to complications in subsequent pregnancies, lead to weight retention throughout life, and contribute to obesity. To date, there is limited information as to the hormonal effects a woman with PCOS will endure during her postpartum period. One study shows that insulin levels remain relatively low postpartum in PCOS women who are lactating compared to pre-pregnancy levels and are similar to those of lactating women without PCOS (62). The authors suggest that lactation can be a "critical period for the improvement of metabolic control" of PCOS women (62) and further supports the benefits of breastfeeding.

Lactation may help women lose weight after childbirth due to increased calories burned (on average, 500 calories per day for a normal weight woman in the first 6 months) as there is a higher demand for glucose by the mammary gland. However, there are many obstacles to self-care that may prevent a woman from being able to lose weight, especially if she is not breastfeeding. One main obstacle is lack of sleep. Anyone reading this with children can relate to the first few months of a baby's life which are accompanied by many sleepless nights! Insufficient sleep is related to weight gain and hormonal changes. In fact, sleep deprivation has been associated with decreased leptin and increased ghrelin, both of which may stimulate hunger and appetite, especially for high carbohydrate and energy dense foods (63). This can be problematic for the PCOS woman as refined foods can worsen insulin levels and lead to weight gain. Additionally, some women may find themselves engaging in binge or emotional eating during sleepless nights when they are up caring for their baby, which can also contribute to weight gain and/or resistance to postpartum weight loss. Registered dietitians can help patients become more aware of their emotional triggers and identify more healthy ways of coping with their emotions other than turning to food for support.

Lack of exercise is another factor contributing to postpartum weight retention. Finding time for physical activity with a newborn can be particularly challenging without proper support. Sampselle et al. studied exercise levels of 1,003 women who were 6 weeks postpartum. Those who reported higher levels of exercise retained significantly less weight after 6 weeks than those who reported less physical activity (64). If possible, it would be beneficial for dietitians working with PCOS women to discuss plans for physical activity after childbirth while pregnant in order to make it a priority. This could include exercising at home, joining exercise classes with their baby, finding areas they can walk with the baby in a stroller or carrier (parks, malls), or deciding who may watch their child during exercise, perhaps utilizing childcare services at gyms.

Dietary changes postpartum are another obstacle. The added responsibility and time demands of caring for a newborn can affect one's ability to make wise food choices and purchase and prepare healthier meals. It could also affect a woman's ability to respond to her own needs for food as she can't always eat when she needs to. According to Debra Krummel, PhD, RD, the first step in providing nutrition counseling to a woman for postpartum weight management is to assess client's readiness, intention, and barriers to change (28). This will help the dietitian and the patient decide what steps need to be followed in order for change to occur. The use of motivational interviewing as well as support from regular follow-up sessions, may help patients to believe they can commit to making healthier changes while caring for a newborn.

During the postpartum period it remains important for PCOS women to be following a diet moderate in whole-grain carbohydrates and lean proteins as it was in pregnancy, whether they are nursing or not, to control insulin and glucose levels. The EAR for carbohydrates during lactation is 160 grams/day, and the Adequate Intake (AI) is 210 grams/day (37). It is equally important to be eating often throughout the day, stressing the need to have sufficient food at home that can easily be prepared and eaten. I advise my PCOS patients who have small children and who are often on the run to always carry snacks in their purse or diaper bag in case they get hungry, just as they provide for their children. Snacks should ideally contain protein and be able to hold up in hot environments, such as nuts. Some of my patients keep a small cooler in the trunks of their cars in which they can add ice packs and food that need refrigeration.

Nutrition professionals can work with patients to determine some quick and easy meals and snacks, and choose healthier alternatives when ordering take-out. Providing patients with a meal plan consisting of appropriate daily caloric amounts and education on portion sizes can be beneficial to postpartum weight loss especially since they may have been accustomed to eating a higher caloric intake during pregnancy. Due to its affect on milk production, it is not advisable for nursing mothers to consume fewer than 1500 calories each day. Dietitians can also encourage patients to accept support from family and friends who want to help in grocery shopping and meal making. Stocking the freezer with frozen foods such as vegetables and healthy homemade meals prepared during pregnancy can also be useful.

In summary, the joyous time of pregnancy can pose some additional concerns to PCOS women as they are at a higher risk for miscarriage and obstetrical complications. Some PCOS women may be resistant to eating carbohydrate foods or consume too much of them, posing additional risks to mother and fetus. Dietitians need to educate patients on the benefits of a good diet and lifestyle to sustain a healthy pregnancy. Dietetic professionals should also provide patients with education on appropriate amounts of weight gain. Women with PCOS may have concerns during the postpartum period that could affect lactation, eating habits, and overall, weight management. MNT, therefore, plays an integral part in the health of PCOS women during pregnancy and throughout the postpartum period.

CHAPTER SUMMARY

- Women with PCOS have higher rates of miscarriage and may be more prone to developing gestational diabetes.
- OGTT should be initiated earlier in PCOS women, at 20 weeks gestation and again at 28 weeks gestation.
- Carbohydrate intake should be 35-40% of total calories with an emphasis on high fiber foods, spread evenly throughout the day.
- Adequate intake of essential fatty acids is necessary during pregnancy and the postpartum period.
- Many herbs and botanicals used by PCOS women are contraindicated during pregnancy.
- Metformin during pregnancy reduces miscarriage, gestational diabetes, pre-eclampsia, macrosomia, and preterm labor in women with PCOS.
- Metformin use in pregnancy has not been proven to affect the growth or motor-social development of infants up to 18 months of life.
- Metformin has been shown to cross into breast milk in "clinically insignificant amounts" and does not appear to cause any adverse health risks in infants up to 6 months of age.

- Hormonal imbalances in PCOS may affect the ability to establish adequate breast development and milk production in nursing moms. Working with a board-certified lactation consultant and the use of herbal or medical treatments may help increase milk supply.
- A number of obstacles can affect postpartum weight loss including sleep depravation, stress, dietary changes, and lack of exercise.

REFERENCES

1. Jakubowicz DJ, Iuorno MJ, Jakubowicz S, et al. Effects of metformin on early pregnancy loss in the polycystic ovary syndrome. *J Clin Endocrinol Metab.* 2002;87:524-529.

2. Seale FG, IV, Robinson RD, Neal GS. Association of metformin and pregnany in the polycystic ovary syndrome: a report of three cases. *J Reprod Med.* 2000;45:507-510.

3. Barbierei RL. Metformin for the treatment of polycystic ovary syndrome. *Obstet Gynedcol.* 2003;101:785-793.

4. Thadhani R, Stampfer MJ, Hunter DJ, Manson JE, Solomon CO, Curhan GC. High body mass index and hypercholesterolemia: risk of hypertensive disorders of pregnancy. *Obstet Gynecol.*1999;'94:543-50.

5. Sarwer D, Allison K, Gibbons L, Tuttman Markowitz J, Nelson DB. Pregnancy and obesity: a review and agenda for future research. *J Women Health.* 2006;15(6):720-733.

6. Siega-Riz A, Laraia B. The implications of maternal overweight and obesity on the course of pregnancy and birth outcomes. *Matern Child Health J.* 2006;10:S153-S156.

7. Hurley KM, Caulfield LE, Sacco LM, Costigan KA, Dipietro JA. Psychosocial influences in dietary patterns during pregnancy. *J Am Diet Assoc.* 2005;105:963.

8. Shabert J. Nutrition during pregnancy and lactation. In: Mahan K, Escott-Stump S. *Krause's Food Nutrition, and Diet Therapy,* 11th ed. Philadelphia PA: Saunders; 2004:183.

9. Thatcher S. Now I'm pregnant. Is the pregnancy at greater risk? Thatcher S. In: *Polycystic Ovary Syndrome: The Hidden Epidemic.* Indianapolis, IN: Perspectives Press; 2007:215-242.

10. Solomon CG, Willett WC, Carey VJ, Rich-Edwards J, Hunter DJ, Colditz GA. A prospective study of pregravid determinants of gestational diabetes mellitus. *JAMA.* 1997;278:1078-83.

11. Anderson JL, Waller DK, Canfield MA, Shaw GM, Watkins ML, Werler MM. Maternal obesity, gestational diabetes, and central nervous system birth defects. *Epidemiology.* 2005;16:87-92.

12. Vahratian A, Siega-Riz AM, Zhang J, Troendle J, Savitz D. Maternal pre-pregnancy overweight and obesity and the risk of primary cesarean delivery in nulliparous women. *Ann Epidemiol.* 2005;15:467-74.

13. Chattingius S, Bergstrom R, Lipworth L, Kramer MS. Prepregnancy weight and the risk of adverse pregnancy outcomes. *N Engl J Med.* 1998;338-147-52.

14. Rosenberg TJ, Barbers S, Chavkin W, Chiasson MA. Prepregnancy weight and adverse perinatal outcomes in an ethnically diverse population. *Obstet Gynecol.* 2003;102;1022-7.

15. Vahratian A, Siega-Riz AM, Zhang J, Troendle J. Maternal pre-pregnancy overweight and obesity and the pattern of labor progression in term nulliparous women. *Obst Gynecol.* 2004.104:943-51.

16. Larsen CE, Serdula MK, Sullivan KM. Macrosomia: influence of maternal overweight among a low-income population. *Am J Obstet Gynecol.* 1990;162:490-94.

17. Haakova L, Cibula D, Rezabeck K, Hill M, Fanta M, Zivny J. Pregnancy outcome in women with PCOS and in controls matched by age and weight. *Human Reproduction.* 2003;18(7):1438-1441.

18. Lanzone A, Fulghesu AM, Cucinelli F, Guido M, Pavone V. Preconceptional and gestational evaluation of insulin secretion in patients with polycystic ovary syndrome. *Hum Reprod.* 1996;11:2382-2386.

19. Mikola M, Hiilesmaa V, halttunen M, Suhonen L, Tittinen A. Obstetric outcome in women with polycystic ovary syndrome. *Hum Reprod.* 2001;16:226-229.

20. Radon PA, McMahon, MJ, Meyer WR. Impaired glucose tolerance in pregnant women with polycystic ovary syndrome. *Obstet Gynecol.*1990;94;194-197.

21. Metzger BE, Coustan DR (Eds.): Proceedings of the Fourth International Work-shop Conference on Gestational Diabetes

Mellitus. *Diabetes Care.* 1998;21(S):B1-B167.

22. American Diabetes Association: Gestational diabetes mellitus [Position statement], *Diabetes Care.* 2004;27:S88-90.

23. Tran N, Hunter S, Yankowitz J. Oral hypoglycemic agents in pregnancy. *Obstetrical and gynecological Survey.* 2004;59(6):456-463.

24. Institute of Medicine, Nutritional status and weight gain. In: *Nutrition during pregnancy.* Wahsington, DC. National Academy Press, 1990;27.

25. Johnson JW, Yancey MK. A critique of the new recommendations for weight gain in pregnancy. *Am J Obstet Gynecol.* 1996;174-254.

26. Feig DS, Naylor CD. Eating for two: are guidelines for weight gain during pregnancy too liberal? *Lancet.* 1998;351-1054.

27. Cogswell ME, Scanlon KS, Fein SB. Medicallyl advised, mother's personal target, and actual weight gain during pregnancy. *Obstet Gynecol.* 1999;94;616.

28. Krummel D. Postpartum weight control: A vicious cycle. *J Am Diet Asso.* 2007;107:37-40.

29. Brawarsky P, Stotland NE, Jackson RA, Fuentes-Afflick E. Pre-pregnancy and pregnancy related factors and the risk of excessive or inadequate gestational weight gain. *Int J Gynecol Obstet.* 2005;91:125-131.

30. Galtier-Dereure F, Boegner C, Bringer J. Obesity and pregnancy: complications and cost. *Am J Clin Nutr.* 2000;71:1242S-1248S.

31. Butte NF, Ellis KJ, Wong WW, Hopkinshon JM, O'Brien Smith E. Composition of gestational weight gain impacts maternal fat retention and infant birth weight. *Am J Obstet Gynecol.* 2003;189:1423-1432.

32. Strauss RS, Dietz WH. Low maternal weight gain in the second or third trimester increases the risk for intrauterine growth retardation. *J Nutr.* 1999;129:988-933.

33. American Dietetic Association: Nutrition and lifestyle for a healthy pregnancy outcome [Position Statement]. *J Amer Diet Assoc.* 2002;102(10): 1479-1490.

34. U.S. Department of Health and Human Services, National Institutes of Health. Healthy eating and physical activity across your life-span: fit for two: tips for pregnancy. NIDDK weight-control information network. NIH Publication.No. 02-5130, 2002.

35. Barker DJP, Hales CN, Fall CHD, Osmond C, Phillips K, Clark PMS. Type 2 (non-insulin-dependent) diabetes mellitus, hypertension,

and hyperlipidemia (syndrome x): relation to reduced fetal growth. *Diabetologia.* 1993;36:62-67.

36. Moses RG, Luebcke L, Davis WS, Coleman KJ,Tapsell LC, Petocz P, Brand-Miller JC. Effect of a low-glycemic-index diet during pregnancy on obstetric care. *Amer J Clin Nut.* 2006;84:807-812.

37. Institute of Medicine, Food and Nutrition Board: *Dietary reference intakes for energy and the macronutrients, carbohydrate, fat, fiber, and fatty acids.* Washington DC, 2002, National Academy Press.

38. Brown JE. Nutrition during pregnancy. In: Brown JE. *Nutrition Through the Lifecycle,* 2nd ed. Belmont, CA: Thompson Wadsworth; 2005:95

39. Scholl TO, Chen X, Khoo CS, Lenders C. The dietary glycemic index during pregnancy: influence on infant birth weight, fetal growth, and biomarkers of carbohydrate. *Am J Epidemiol.* 2004;159:467-474.

40. Zhang C, Liu S, Solomon C, Hu F. Dietary fiber intake, dietary glycemic load, and the risk for gestational diabetes mellitus. *Diabetes Care.* 2006;29(10):2223-2230.

41. Sanders T. Essential fatty acid requirements of vegetarians in pregnancy, lactation, and infancy *Amer J of Clin Nut.* 1999;70(3)3:555S-559S.

42. Hornstra G. Essential fatty acids in mothers and their neonates. *Amer J Clinic Nutr.* 2000;71(5): 1262S-1269S.

43. Carlson SE, Werkman SH, Peeples JM, Wilson WE. Long-chain fatty acids and early visual and cognitive development of preterm infants. *Eur J Clin Nutr.* 1994;48(suppl):27–30.

44. American Academy Pediatrics, Committee on Nutrition. *Pediatric Nutrition Handbook.* Elk Grove Village, IL: American Academy Pediatrics;1998.

45. Foote J, Rengers B. Maternal use of herbal supplements. *Nutrition in Complementary Care.* 2000;1.

46. Cartwright, MM. Herbal use during pregnancy and lactation: a need for caution. The Digest 2001;(Summer):1-3. American Dietetic Association Public Health/Community Nutrition Practice Group.

47. *Nutrition and Your Health: Dietary Guidelines for Americans.* 5th ed. Washington, DC: US Departments of Agriculture and Health and Human Services. 2000. Home and Garden Bulletin No.232.

48. Sirtori CR, Pasik C. Re-evaluation of a biguanide, metformin:

mechanism of action and tolerability. *Pharmacol Res.*1994;30:187-228.

49. Langner O. When diet fails: insulin and oral hypoglycemic agents as alternatives for the management of gestational diabetes mellitus. *J Matern Fetal Neonatal Med.* 2002;11:218-225.

50. Glueck C, Goldenberg N, Pranikoff J, Loftspring M, Sieve L, Wang P. Height, weight, and motor-social development during the first 18 months of life in 126 infants born to 109 mothers with poly-cystic ovary syndrome who conceived on and continued metformin through pregnancy. *Human Reproduction.* 2004;19(6):1323-1330.

51. Marasco, L. *Insufficient milk supply: Common Factors and Relationship to Polycystic Ovary Syndrome.* Master's thesis. Pacific Oaks College, Pasadena, CA;2001.

52. Lisa Marasco, MA, IBCLC, personal communication, March 2007.

53. Marasco L, Marmet C, Shell E. Polycystic Ovary Syndrome: A connection to insufficient milk supply? *Journal of Human Lactation* 2000;16(2):143-148.

54. Strode MA, Dewey KG, Lonnerdal B. Effects of short-term caloric restricition on lactational performance of well-nourished women. *Acta Paediatr Scand.* 1986;75(2):222-9.

55. Hardy ML. Herbs of special interest to women. *J Amer Pharm Assoc.* 2000;40:2234.

56. Briggs G, Ambrose P, Nagcotte M, Padilla G, Wan S. Excretion of metformin into breast milk and the effect on nursing infants. *Obstet Gynecol* 2005;105:1437-41.

57. Hale TW, Kristensen JH, Hackett LP, Kohan R, Ilett KF. Transfer of metformin into human milk. *Diabetologia* 2002;45:1509-1514.

58. Gardiner S, Kirkpatrick C, Begg E, Zhang M, Moore MP, Saville D. Transfer of metformin into human milk. *Clin Pharmacol Ther* 2003;73:71-7.

59. Glueck C, Salehi M, Sieve L, Wang P. Growth, motor, and social development in breast-and formula-fed infants of metformin treated women with polycystic ovary syndrome. *J Pediatr* 2006;148:628-32.

60. Rooney BL, Schauberger CW. Excess pregnancy weight gain and long-term obesity: one decade later. *Obstet Gynecol.* 2002;100:245.

61. Linney, Dye L, Barkeling B, Rossner S. Long-term weight develop-ment in women: a 15-year follow up of the effects of pregnancy. *Obes Res.* 2004;12:1116.

62. Maliqueo M, Sir-Petermann t, Salazaar G, Bravo F, Wildt L. Resumption of ovarian function during lactational amenorrhoea in breastfeeding women with polycystic ovarian syndrome: metabolic aspects. *Human Reproduction.* 2001;16(8):1598-1602.
63. Taheri S, Lin L, Austin d, Young T, Mignot E. Short sleep duration is associated with reduced leptin, elevated ghrelin, and increased body mass index. *PLoS Med.* 2004;1:e62.
64. Sampselle CM, Seng J, Yeo S, Killion C, Oakley D. Physical activity and postpartum well-being. *J Obstet Gynecol Neonatal Nurs.* 1999;28:41.

CHAPTER 8

PCOS AND EATING DISORDERS

THE FIRST TIME I heard of polycystic ovary syndrome (PCOS) was in 1999 while working for an eating disorder treatment facility. A patient named Sarah, age 27, tearfully explained to me the symptoms that she was experiencing: severe acne and hair growth on her face, absent periods, thinning hair, and her weight had been increasing almost two pounds each month for the past year. She hated her body and felt it was out of control. She had just been diagnosed with PCOS three weeks earlier and her doctor recommended that she try the Atkins carbohydrate-free diet to manage her insulin and help her to lose weight. Through the tears, Sarah admitted that she had tried to follow the diet but that she just kept bingeing on carbohydrates and felt so guilty afterwards that she purged to get rid of them. Sarah also had a long history of bulimia nervosa.

MENSTRUAL DISTURBANCES

It is widely accepted that women with eating disorders, whether it be from anorexia nervosa (AN), bulimia nervosa (BN) or a combination of several symptoms of eating disorders commonly referred to as eating disorder not otherwise specified (EDNOS), have menstrual disturbances (1-3). Much like women with PCOS, these menstrual disturbances include anovulation and oligomenorrhea (menstrual cycles longer than 40 days) (4).

In a recent study, researchers examined the hormonal dysfunctions associated with improper eating habits among 14 subjects with BN and 22 subjects with EDNOS (4). They found decreased levels of follicle stimulating hormone (FSH) and lutenizing hormone (LH) among both groups with the EDNOS group having the lowest levels of the two hormones and higher amounts of testosterone than controls. The researchers suggest that one reason why many women with BN and EDNOS may have menstrual disturbances is related to low levels of LH, which is a sensitive variant affected by dramatic changes in eating habits (4). Thus, crash dieting or restricting, common bulimic and compulsive eating behaviors may affect levels of LH. This can result in an insufficient luteal phase, producing oligomenorrhea or anovulation seen in PCOS.

THE EMOTIONAL TOLL

Like my patient Sarah, the symptoms many women with PCOS endure can have a direct effect on their body image and self-esteem and it may lead to the development of distorted eating habits or eating disorders, linking the two conditions (5). There seems to be a genetic component to the development of PCOS with studies indicating that some girls are even born with cysts on their ovaries (6). Most symptoms, however, do not appear until the onset of puberty - another factor in common with eating disorders. For example, right at a time when a young woman's self-esteem is quite vulnerable, she may start to experience acne and excessive hair growth on her face and other parts of her body along with weight gain in her mid-section, setting her apart from her peers. Not knowing that she has PCOS or why her body is reacting in the way that it is, she may begin to blame herself and hate her body. Struggling with these issues at such a vulnerable time can lead many young women to deal with their emotional distress through unhealthy dieting practices such as laxatives, diuretics and diet pills, fasting, and engaging in excessive exercise and vomiting. These negative behaviors can set the stage for a lifetime of eating issues and body hatred.

Researchers have investigated the relationship between monozygotic and dizygotic twins with PCOS and BN by using the BITE questionnaire (Bulimia Investigation Test, Edinburgh), a self-rating scale used to diagnose BN that includes 30 questions about dieting and binge behaviors such as "does your pattern of eating severely disrupt your life?," "do you ever experience overpowering urges to eat and eat?" and "do you ever fast for a whole day?" (7). They found that 76% of PCOS twins had elevated scores on the BITE, suggesting that a relationship does in fact exist between BN and PCOS. Other studies conducted using the BITE questionnaire support a relationship between PCOS and binge eating with one-third of women with PCOS in one study demonstrating binge eating behavior (8).

The development of binge eating among PCOS women is all too common. Many women with PCOS are very frustrated and fed-up with their diagnosis. They feel immense pressure because they desperately want to lose weight, conceive a child, and overall improve their symptoms; they believe the only way to do this is by dieting. Often times they will restrict carbohydrates in order to lose weight or sometimes they eat limited amounts of food. This, combined with their carbohydrate cravings and hypoglycemia, result in bingeing and feeling even worse about themselves. After consuming large amounts of food and feeling the guilt associated with a binge, they tend to want to restrict their intake, purge, or engage in other unhealthy behaviors to get rid of the overwhelming feelings. This in turn, can set them up for another binge episode. Thus a vicious cycle ensues.

On the other hand, many women with PCOS have a long history of yo-yo dieting. Even before knowing they had PCOS they struggled with their weight, either trying to prevent the number on the scale from creeping up or trying to make it go down, only to lose weight and gain it back. The result of being on so many different types of diets, each time looking for a quick fix, is that they learn to view foods as "good" or "bad". Therefore, they feel guilty if they eat certain "bad" foods and in turn, feel bad about themselves. They also learn not to trust their bodies as to when they need food, how much food they need, and whether or not they need it.

In addition, it is known that women with PCOS, because of their hormonal imbalances, may be more prone to mood swings and depression than someone without PCOS. Having elevated testosterone may in fact make women with PCOS more aggressive, angry, anxious, and depressed. Many women with PCOS, however, may also have mood disturbances from having to deal with the symptoms associated with their diagnosis (9). As discussed in Chapter 2, co-diagnosis of mental health problems is very common among individuals with eating disorders. Some clients may benefit from consulting with a psychiatrist to assess the use of anti-depressants or anti-anxiety medications in addition to regularly working with a therapist.

THE INSULIN EFFECT

It is understandable that women with PCOS may become more susceptible to developing an eating disorder and suffer from body image disturbances, but can women with eating disorders develop PCOS?

It has been proposed that insulin may have an appetite stimulating effect and can perpetuate binge behavior (1). For example, during an eating binge when large quantities of food are consumed over a relatively short amount of time, there is a surge of excess insulin, much more than experienced during a normal meal. Constant bingeing could, therefore, result in a chronic state of elevated insulin. Hyperinsulinemia stimulates the ovaries to produce more androgens (1). As a result, women with PCOS who engage in binge eating will further increase insulin levels and cause a worsening of their PCOS symptoms.

Researchers have investigated whether women with bulimia are insulin resistant and examined the relationship between insulin and androgen levels, ovarian morphology and severity of bulimic behavior (1). Although they did not find that women with bulimia had insulin resistance, they did find that they were chronically hyperinsulinemic with 10 of their 12 normal weight subjects having polycystic ovaries (4). This led the researchers to speculate that hyperinsulinemia may be one of the reasons why a connection exists between bulimia and PCOS. The bulimic pattern of bingeing followed by starvation and/or vomiting perpetuates the insulin response and leads to the development of polycystic ovaries (1). It may also suggest why some women who are overweight or obese without a family history develop PCOS through overfeeding.

There is some encouraging news: it appears that when women

with PCOS and bulimia return to normalized eating patterns with treatment involving cognitive behavioral therapy (CBT), it can result in improved ovarian morphology (3). Chronic bingeing can worsen the appearance of polycystic ovaries but ovarian morphology does seem to resolve when binging ceases and normal eating patterns are established.

IMPAIRED APPETITE REGULATION

New research suggests that women who have PCOS also have impaired secretion of the hormone cholecystokinin (CCK) resulting in a reduced feeling of satiety (10). CCK is released from the small intestine in response to the presence of food and plays an important role in regulating appetite. It has been previously believed that women with BN also have impaired CCK secretion (11) and could also explain the tendencies of women with PCOS, BN or EDNOS to crave sweets, binge eat or be overweight because of their impaired ability to feel fullness. It is not known why women with PCOS have impaired CCK secretion following meals, but it has been suggested that like individuals with BN and diabetes, women with PCOS may have delayed gastric emptying (10).

Impaired levels of leptin and ghrelin have also been documented in PCOS (12), further suggesting that women with PCOS have dysfunctional appetite regulation. Fasting levels of ghrelin, the stomach-derived hormone that is secreted to signal hunger, has been found to be impaired in lean and obese women with PCOS compared to weight matched non-PCOS women (12). In one study, overweight subjects with PCOS were less satiated and hungrier after test meals than overweight subjects without PCOS (12).

Furthermore, it has been documented that leptin, a protein hormone involved in energy balance that is secreted to signal satiety, is also compromised in PCOS women (13). A positive correlation exists between leptin and BMI and between leptin and testosterone in women with PCOS (13). Decreased leptin function may stimulate feeding in PCOS women, resulting in increased food intake and difficulties managing weight (14). In addition, having impaired levels of CCK and gherilin could also explain why PCOS women are resistant to weight loss since appetite signals are compromised, making them hungrier and wanting to eat more.

Interestingly, a relationship has been documented between between leptin, subclinical eating disorders, and PCOS (14). Leptin concentrations in women with AN have been found to be lower than those of normal-weight controls (15). Leptin may even be implicated in the pathophysiology of PCOS as it is also involved in reproductive function (16).

NUTRITION MANAGEMENT FOR THE PCOS WOMAN WITH DISTORTED EATING

The most commonly agreed upon recommendations to improve insulin levels and reproductive function in PCOS are eating a diet that is lower in carbohydrates with an emphasis on low-glycemic index (GI) foods and regular exercise (17). However, because women with PCOS may be more prone to binge eating, it is imperative that dietitians screen patients with PCOS for eating disorders before recommending dieting or changes in eating behavior. Effective questions to ask during the initial assessment include:

- "Tell me how you feel about your weight."
- "Describe your control of food."
- "What types of foods do you feel out of control with?"
- "Tell me about your feelings of hunger and fullness."
- "How do you feel about eating foods containing carbohydrates?"
- "Tell me about any methods you use to control your weight."
- "How do you feel when you eat with other people?"
- "How do you feel when you eat, while doing something else at the same time (i.e., in front of the TV or computer)?"

If distorted eating is suspected, the first focus should be on normalizing eating patterns to control insulin levels and prevent bingeing and weight gain. Even without focusing on weight loss, ovarian morphology and insulin levels may improve by the restoration of normal eating patterns (3). Many of the physicians I work with prefer to monitor clients' insulin and hemoglobin A1-C (HA1C) levels (in addition to liver function tests) approximately every 3 months. This can be a valuable measure to reflect changes in the clients' eating. It can also be a useful motivating tool to show a client that although they may not have lost weight, the positive changes they have made in their eating have resulted in reduced insulin levels and overall improvement in their health.

Clients need to be educated on the importance of structuring regular meals and snacks throughout the day to stabilize blood sugar levels and prevent cravings and hypoglycemic episodes. This may include eating every 3-5 hours with the addition of at least 1 to 2 protein exchanges with meals and snacks (17). Protein adds to satiety and delays the release of glucose, acting as a buffer to manage insulin levels. Some clients may benefit from pre-planning their meals and snacks ahead of time; this can reduce anxiety and give the client a better sense of comfort, knowing that more food is available later. In addition, I have noticed that many of my clients with PCOS who take insulin-lowering medications such as metformin report little or no hypoglycemic episodes, less carbohydrate cravings, and reduced interest in food overall.

Weight loss is very difficult among women with PCOS as they may have to cut back drastically in comparison to their peers in order to achieve any weight loss. Because of their struggles in maintaining weight through dieting, many women with PCOS may have lost their internal ability to regulate food intake. For example, they may not be able to effectively distinguish when they are hungry. This could result in them eating when they don't need to or waiting long periods to eat. If they do use food to cope with emotions, perhaps they are unable to distinguish when they are physically satisfied with food leading them to eat more than they need to. Part of establishing life-long normalized eating patterns should, therefore, involve education on self-care and mindful eating.

FOOD LOGS

The use of food logs to rate hunger and satisfaction levels before and after meals can be a very effective technique for promoting self-awareness. I encourage my clients to use a scale from 0 to 10 with 0 being completely starving, 5 neutral (not hungry or full), and 10 being "Thanksgiving dinner stuffed". They are to check in with themselves at various times throughout the day to assess their number and especially before, during, and after meals to determine when they need food and how much.

Most women who have kept food logs in the past either for various diet plans or for their own self use, have not monitored their hunger or satiety levels before. Checking their hunger and satiety can be very difficult, almost seeming impossible at first to the PCOS woman who has been a chronic dieter for most of her life. It is important to let the client know that it may be difficult for her to do this at first, but it is a process that she must practice and experiment with to eventually be able to listen and respond to her internal cues. Reviewing the logs together can help clients identify when they are eating when they do not need to, if they ate for emotional reasons, or if they ate enough food at the meal to feel satisfied that it could hold them over until the next time they ate. This also provides a great opportunity to explore and challenge client's attitudes toward food and weight.

CONSCIOUS EATING EXERCISES

I like to use conscious eating exercises with my clients in nutrition sessions that they can also practice at home. This would mean eating food together either as a meal or a snack, and consciously recognize how the food tastes and feels to them (I have even done this by using a single cracker, raisin, grape, or piece of chocolate). These exercises can be extremely beneficial to the PCOS woman who often eats on the run, eats while standing, or eats in front of her TV or computer screen. Usually, when people eat while they are doing something like watching TV or driving, they have to focus on what is in front of them and therefore, are not focusing on tasting the food. After completing the conscious eating exercise, I will ask clients how it feels to eat mindfully rather than eating while being distracted by something. It really is an eye-opening exercise.

I discuss mindful eating exercises with clients at preceding sessions so that they are prepared and remember to bring their food to subsequent planned sessions (I always keep snacks in my office too). I bring my own food and usually eat with my clients; I find it to be a great way to model mindful eating and it makes the client feel more comfortable than having to eat by themselves.

To begin a mindful eating or conscious eating exercise in a nutrition session, I first start by having the client set up their food, drink, and utensils on the table. Next I lead them through a relaxation exercise or encourage deep breathing. We will then begin by having the client examine the food that they brought by observing the color, shape, and texture. The next step is for the client to pick up part of their food and, if they can, feel it for its texture. Finally, I instruct the client to place the bite of food (or whole grape or cracker) in their mouth, noting the feel and texture of that food prior to chewing. They can then start slowly chewing the food and swallowing, again noting any feelings or sensations they experience when they do this. The client repeats the exercise by eating mindfully with each bite of food they take. They are encouraged to practice this outside of nutrition sessions by using their food logs to rate their degree of hunger and satisfaction levels before and after meals. To effectively practice these exercises, eating should be done in a relaxed setting at a table away from distractions of work, the computer, and TV.

CHALLENGING NEGATIVE THOUGHTS

Because of their history with dieting, many women with PCOS may have some negative and false beliefs about food. Some of these beliefs you may hear include the following statements: "I can't eat any foods that contain carbohydrates," "carbs are bad," "I can't eat fruit because they are all carbs," or "fat is bad." As dietitians, it is part of our role to provide objective and reliable nutrition information to the public and clear up any false beliefs, especially if it has a direct effect on a client's health. For example, educating your client that fruit contains carbohydrates. However, it is unhealthy for a woman with PCOS to avoid fruit because the nutrients in it are beneficial in fighting cancer, preventing hypertension and constipation, plus they help you feel physically satisfied.

Carbohydrates may be especially fearful to the PCOS woman who has been told perhaps by her physician or the internet to limit all carbs from her diet. This is very problematic to someone with a history of an eating disorder or, as discussed earlier, can lead to the development of an eating disorder. It may be in the client's best interest to try and include some form of a whole grain carbohydrate source at each meal or snack at first to help the client break out of a binge or binge-purge cycle, regulate blood sugar levels and control for hypoglycemia. Some clients are fearful that if they add carbohydrates back into their diets that they will lose control and start bingeing on them. In this case, clients should add carbohydrates gradually, starting with those that are "safest" to them. Clients need to know from the nutrition expert that it is ok to eat carbohydrates again; they will need regular reassurance of why it may be beneficial to include carbohydrates in a healthy diet. It is also helpful to check in regularly with your client to see how they are feeling about having some carbohydrate sources at meals or snacks and if they think it benefits them to do so.

COPING SKILLS

Most of all, women struggling with PCOS and eating disorders need to learn effective ways to deal with their emotions without abusing food. Dietitians can help clients identify possible alternative coping skills other than food and should support clients to apply these new skills into their lives. For example, I will have my clients make a list of positive things they can do when they have urges to binge. This may include activities such as taking a walk, reading, journaling, calling a friend, surfing the internet or taking a bath. Clients are encouraged to try and apply some of the activities on the list to overcome urges and find the ones that work best for them. In addition, working with a psychotherapist may help individuals identify their emotional triggers and encourage mindfulness and behavior change.

Once normalized eating patterns have been established and clients are able to respond to internal cues of hunger and satiety without using eating disorder symptoms, further recommendations on diet and exercise may be advised with caution and should focus on continuing to improve overall health rather than weight loss (18,19).

CHAPTER SUMMARY

- Like women with PCOS, women who have eating disorders also tend to have high rates of menstrual disturbances.
- Erratic eating habits, such as periods of restricting followed by bingeing and/or purging, can have a hormonal effect and cause menstrual disturbances.
- Women with PCOS are at a higher risk for developing an eating disorder or distorted eating because of the detrimental effects of their symptoms on body image, weight, and mood disturbances.
- Insulin has an appetite stimulating effect and may make PCOS women more prone to binge eating, especially when engaging in restrictive eating.
- PCOS women have impaired secretion of cholecystokinin, leptin, and ghrelin, thus affecting appetite regulation.
- It is imperative that dietitians screen patients with PCOS for eating disorders first, before recommending dieting or changes in eating behavior.
- If distorted eating is suspected, the first focus should be on normalizing eating patterns to control insulin levels and prevent bingeing and weight gain.
- Even without focusing on weight loss, ovarian morphology and insulin levels may improve by the restoration of normal eating patterns.
- Dietitians can help clients normalize their eating by providing conscious eating exercises, coping skills, cognitive restructuring techniques and reality checks.

REFERENCES

1. Raphael FJ, Rodin DA, Peattie A, Bano G, Kent A, Nussey SS, Lacey JH. Ovarian morphology and insulin sensitivity in women with bulimia nervosa. *Clinical Endocrinology.* 1995;43:451-5.

2. Michelmore KF, Balen AH, Dunger DB. Polycystic ovaries and eating disorders: are they related? *Human Reproduction.* 2001;16(4):765-769.

3. Morgan J, McCluskey S, Brunton JN, Lacey JH. Polycystic ovarian

morphology and bulimia nervosa: a 9-year follow-up study. *Fert and Sterility.* 2002;77:928-31.

4.   Resch M, Szendei G, Haasz P. Bulimia from a gynecological view: hormonal changes. J of *Obstetrics and Gynaecology.* 2004;24(8):907-910.

5.   McCluskey S, Evans C, Lacey H, Pearce JM, Jacobs H. Polycystic ovary syndrome and bulimia. *Fertil Steril.* 1991;55(2):287-91.

6.   Bridges, NA, Cooke A, Healy M.J, Hindmarsh PC, Brook CG. Standards for ovarian volume in childhood and puberty. *Fertil Steril.* 1993;60:456-460.

7.   Jahanfar S, Eden A, Nguyent TV. Bulimia nervosa and polycystic ovary syndrome. *Gynecol. Endocrinology.* 1995;9:113-7.

8.   McCluskey S, Lacey JH, Pearce JM. Binge-eating and polycystic ovaries. *Lancet.* 1992;340:723.

9.   Weiner C, Primeau M, Ehrmann A. Androgens and mood dysfunction in women: comparison of women with polycystic ovarian syndrome to healthy controls. *Psychosomatic Med.* 2004;66:356-61.

10. Hirschberg AL, Nassen S, Stridsberg M, Bystrom B, Holte J. Impaired cholecystokinin secretion and disturbed appetite regulation in women with polycystic ovary syndrome. *Gynecol Endocrinol.* 2004;19:79-87.

11. Geraciotti TD, Liddle RA. Impaired cholecystokinin secretion in bulimia nervosa. N *Engl J Med.* 1988;319:683-8.

12. Moran LJ, Noakes M, Vlifton PM. Ghrelin and measures of satiety are altered in polycystic ovary syndrome but not differently affected by diet composition. *J Clin Endo and Metabolism.* 2004;893:337-3344.

13. Baranowska B, Radzikowska M, Wasilewska-Dziubinska E, Kaplinski A. Neuropeptide Y, leptin, galanin and insulin in women with polycystic ovary syndrome. *Gynecol Endocrinol.* 1999;13:344-351.

14. Jahanfar S, Malelki H, Mosavi AR. Subclinical eating disorder, polycystic ovary syndrome-is there any connection between these two conditions through leptin-a twin study. *Med J Malaysia.* 2005;60(4):441-6).

15. Chan JL, Mantzoros CS. Role of leptin in energy-deprivation states: normal human physiology and clinical implications for hypothalamic amenorrhoea and anorexia nervosa. *Lancet.* 2005;366(9479):74-85.

16. Cervero A, Dominguez F, Horcajadas J. The role of leptin in reproduction. Curr Opin

17. Marsh K, Brand-Miller J. The optimal diet for women with polycystic ovary syndrome? *British J Med.* 2005;94:154-165.

18. Morgan JF. Bulimic eating patterns should be stabilized in polycystic ovarian syndrome. *BMJ.* 1999;318:328.

19. Moran L, Norman R J. Understanding and managing disturbances in insulin metabolism and body weight in women with polycystic ovary syndrome. *Clinical Obstetrics and Gynaecology.* 2004;18(5):719-736.

CHAPTER 9

CASE STUDIES

BY ANGELA GRASSI, MS, RD, LDN
AND
LYNN MONAHAN COUCH, MPH, RD, LDN

THIS CHAPTER DISCUSSES THREE separate case studies in which medical nutrition therapy was provided to clients diagnosed with polycystic ovary syndrome. The first client, Teresa, is a case in which the client originally came in for weight loss and a diet to help increase fertility, only to become pregnant throughout the course of treatment. Her dietary goals had separate foci and challenges. The second case study involves an adolescent, Jamie, who began nutrition counseling for weight loss. I suspected she had PCOS due to several signs and symptoms she revealed during the nutrition assessment. Jamie also struggled with binge eating. Therefore, nutrition strategies involved helping her normalize her eating while improving her health. Finally, the third case involves an obese woman who presented with many adverse health conditions associated with her PCOS. Medical nutrition therapy interventions focused on helping her change her eating and lifestyle behaviors to prevent the onset of diabetes and to reduce her risk for heart disease.

CASE 1

Teresa was a 27 year-old woman who first came to see me in January for a nutrition assessment. Teresa had a miscarriage of triplets 8 months earlier. She was diagnosed with PCOS one year ago by a reproductive endocrinologist who referred her for nutrition counseling. Teresa wanted help losing weight and improving her diet in hopes it would increase her chances of conceiving again. Also, she wanted to do what she could nutritionally to carry her next pregnancy to term.

Teresa had been married for 1 year and worked in customer service at a department store. She did not exercise, stating that she was on her feet all day and was exhausted when she got home. She did, however, say she knew it was important for her to exercise for weight loss and to improve her PCOS.

She was 5'6" and weighed 245 pounds, her highest weight ever. She reported that her weight had been stable for the past 2 years and she was always overweight growing up. Teresa struggled with other PCOS symptoms of excessive hair growth on her face, inner thighs, and belly button areas. She treated it by electrolysis. Her periods were always irregular, occurring every few months, and were heavy and accompanied by clots. She also had acne and experienced symptoms of hypoglycemia. Her pertinent lab results are shown in table 1.

Table I. Lab results for Teresa

Lab Test	Results	Normal Ranges	Significance
Insulin (fasting)	22	<10 mIU/L	↑ insulin resistance
TSH	0.1.6	0.40 – 5.50 uIU/mL	WNL
Albumin	4.0	3.7-6.1 g/dL	WNL
Total Testosterone	82	8-63 ng/dL (ideal <50)	↑ hyperandrogenism
HbAIC	5.5	<6.0%	WNL
Glucose (fasting)	87	70 – 99 mg/dL	WNL
Total Cholesterol	210	<200 mg/dL	↑ hypercholesterolemia
LDL Cholesterol	183	<130 mg/dL	↑ hypercholesterolemia

Triglycerides	250	<150 mg/dL	↑ hypertriglyceridemia

She had been taking 850 mg of metformin daily for the past month and experienced diarrhea. Her physician wanted her to work up to 2,000 mg daily, however, she was resistant to taking more as she was not comfortable leaving her position at work to go to the bathroom often. She also took 125 mg of clomid. Besides PCOS, Teresa had dyslipidemia. No other medical complications were reported. Her 24-hour recall is presented below:

24-hour food recall:
Snack (7am): 1 cup soymilk, "to take the pills with."

Breakfast (10am): 1 cup plain noodles or a peanut butter and jelly (PBJ) sandwich on white bread or a muffin; consumed at work.

Lunch (1-2 pm): 8 oz. can of clam chowder or PBJ sandwich and popcorn or take out Chinese or pizza (2 slices); consumed at work.

Snack (3 pm): chips, a candy bar, or cupcake. "I need something sweet in the afternoon."

Dinner (7-9pm): vegetables and 7-9 oz. meat or breaded and fried fish with 1 ½ cups corn

Snack (10pm): 1 ½ cups of ice cream (2 x/week)

Diet analysis (using mypyramidtracker.gov): 2400 calories, 89 grams (15%) protein, 272 grams (45%) carbohydrate, 19 grams fiber, 107 grams (40%) fat, 38 grams saturated fat, 40 grams monounsaturated, 21 polyunsaturated, 16.4 grams linoleic acid, 1.6 alpha-linolenic acid, 250 grams cholesterol, 3410 grams sodium.

She reported consuming 48 oz. of water and 12 oz. of regular soda daily. She stated she drank 48 oz. of regular soda and 32 oz. of juice two weeks prior to our assessment. She does not drink alcohol or smoke. In the past she said she ate for emotional reasons but denies doing this now. She also denied any self-induced vomiting, laxatives, diuretics, or diet pill use.

Teresa consumed a very high intake of refined carbohydrates and saturated fat. She consumed limited amounts of vegetables and no fruit. Her sodium intake was also high. Because of her dyslipidemia and insulin resistance, she would benefit from a diet higher in mono and polyunsaturated fatty acids and limited in saturated fat. She also needed to decrease her total carbohydrate intake slightly, replacing refined carbohydrates foods for whole grain.

After completing the assessment of dietary intake, Teresa and I discussed PCOS, including the hormonal imbalances and the role of insulin in the body. I informed Teresa that PCOS women are at an increased risk of miscarriage due to hormonal imbalances, especially because of elevated insulin levels. I also encouraged her to continue taking metformin, working up to her prescribed dosage. Metformin would benefit Teresa by improving ovulation and may be used throughout pregnancy to control insulin levels and to prevent miscarriage. Teresa said she wished she took metformin during her first pregnancy with triplets to possibly prevent her miscarriage.

During this first visit, we discussed how food affects glucose and insulin levels and the differences between refined and whole grain foods. Teresa was able to identify foods in her diet that may have contributed to her hyperinsulinemia. Teresa was also educated on the importance of eating more often throughout the day with protein at every meal and snack. We also discussed the benefits of a small amount of weight loss to improve her reproductive function. Teresa said she was willing to decrease some of her carbohydrates to achieve this.

Teresa's initial nutrition goals were to:
1. Eliminate regular soda.
2. Eat every 3-5 hours with protein at all meals and snacks.
3. Substitute refined carbohydrates with whole grain sources.
4. Decrease carbohydrate intake overall (specifically, she agreed to not bread fish and eat eggs for breakfast at home instead of carbohydrates).
5. Take a prenatal supplement with omega-3 fatty acids daily.

Follow-up session (1 month later)

Teresa happily reported that she thought she was pregnant! She reported following the nutrition goals set at the initial session to control her insulin levels, as she is nervous about possible miscarriage after the loss of her triplets. She is still only taking 850 mg of metformin per day as she says taking more gives her nausea and diarrhea. She is taking a prenatal vitamin daily. She has not been doing any exercise and says she is extremely tired. Teresa also reported a weight loss of 5 pounds since we last met. She said she felt a lot better eating often and having protein with her meals and snacks as she does not experience cravings for sweets or hypoglycemic episodes as before. Below is her 24-hour recall at this follow-up session:

24-hour food recall:
Breakfast (10am): 2 eggs with 1 oz. cheese

Lunch (2pm): grilled cheese sandwich on whole wheat bread, yogurt or milk, fruit

Snack (4pm): ½ cup low-fat cottage cheese and fruit

Dinner (7pm): 7-9 oz. grilled fish, ½ cup broccoli, 1 cup corn,

Snack (9pm): 8 oz. steamed milk

Diet analysis: 1550 calories, 90 grams (23%) protein, 156 grams (38%) carbohydrate, 26 grams fiber, 70 grams (40%) fat, 24 grams saturated, 23 grams monounsaturated, 12 grams polyunsaturated, 10.5 grams linoleic acid, 1.1 grams alpha-linolenic acid, 600 grams cholesterol, 3500 grams sodium.

Teresa's caloric intake was significantly reduced as was her carbohydrate intake. While her total and saturated fat intake decreased, her cholesterol intake increased as Teresa chose foods high in cholesterol (eggs, cheese) as some of her protein sources. Sodium intake was also high.

Teresa made progress in her eating. She ate often and included protein with her meals and snacks. She stopped drinking regular soda and would dilute juice with water. Mostly she was able to eliminate sweets and simple sugars from her diet, substituting refined carbohydrates for whole grain versions.

We discussed the benefits of maintaining a moderate amount of carbohydrates and calories during her first trimester to help manage insulin levels and prevent miscarriage. The importance of eating whole grain carbohydrates was reiterated. Appropriate weight gain ranges during pregnancy were also discussed. Teresa did not know that it was appropriate to maintain her weight during her first (or even second) trimester and that she did not have to "eat for two." The benefits of exercise during pregnancy were also discussed. Teresa was advised to see me at 10 weeks gestation to make further modifications in her eating to support a healthy pregnancy.

Teresa's goals:
1. Maintain current diet of moderate amounts of whole grain carbohydrates during first trimester, limiting refined ones.
2. Use exercise bike for 1 hour, 2 days per week.
3. Continue to work on increasing dosage of metformin.
4. Follow-up nutrition session at 10 weeks gestation.

Second follow-up session (2 months later)
At this visit, Teresa was 15 weeks pregnant (one fetus). She continued to take 850 mg of metformin in addition to her prenatal multivitamin each day. She experienced "horrible" morning sickness and diarrhea in the past 2 months and had lost some more weight. She reported her weight as 238 pounds. Teresa said protein foods, especially fish, poultry, and peanut butter did not appeal to her and she avoided eating them. She did not do any exercise as she reported being tired a lot. Below is her 24-hour recall for this session:

24-hour food recall:
Breakfast (9:30am): 2 cups fruit such as watermelon and pineapple; or she may have a bagel and cream cheese

Lunch (12pm): cheese sandwich on whole wheat with 4 oz. cheese and 16 oz. juice

Snack (3pm): candy bar or whole wheat crackers

Dinner (6pm): steamed crab legs and 16 oz. regular soda.

Diet analysis: 1200 calories, 41 grams protein, 186 grams carbohydrate, 9 grams fiber, 35 grams fat, 20 grams saturated fat, 693 mg sodium.

Teresa was not eating enough protein or calories for pregnancy. She was also consuming a higher amount of simple carbohydrates. Again, I discussed the importance of having sufficient protein with all meals and snacks. I also reinforced the importance of consuming a low GI diet that limited simple sugars. To prevent gestational diabetes mellitus (GDM), it would benefit her if her carbohydrate intake was 35-40% of total calories. Food exchanges were provided. Teresa needed to increase her intake to prevent further weight loss. Together, we made several days worth of sample daily menus. She agreed to keep food logs, recording her degree of hunger and satisfaction with meals.

Teresa's Goals:
1. Increase intake by eating protein-rich foods (that were appealing) with all meals and snacks. Eat eggs or milk with her fruit in the morning and cheese and crackers instead of a candy bar in the afternoon.
2. Limit sweetened beverages to one 8 oz. glass each day.
3. Substitute whole grain carbohydrates over refined ones, staying within recommended amounts.
4. Keep food records, graphing hunger and satiety levels with meals.
5. She was to follow-up with me in 2 weeks to assess diet and weight status.

Third follow-up session (1 month later)

Teresa reported feeling much better and having a better appetite. She was no longer as tired or nauseous. At 19 weeks gestation, Teresa had gained some weight. She reported her weight as 240 pounds. She continued taking 850 grams daily of metformin and her prenatal vitamin. She reported eating more often and making sure to have protein with all her meals and snacks. Food logs were reviewed together. Teresa had limited the refined foods we discussed at previous sessions but was still drinking 16 oz. of regular soda daily. She did not do any exercise. We continued to discuss the importance of eating a low GI diet and exercise in managing insulin levels.

Teresa's Goals:
1. Continue to eat a diet comprised of 35-40% carbohydrates, almost all from whole grain sources, spread evenly throughout the day.
2. Limit sweetened beverages to one 8 oz. glass each day.
3. Have OGTT done within the next 2 weeks to screen early for GDM.
4. Follow-up with me in 1 month to assess diet and weight status.

In the first session, Teresa was very motivated to improve her health and do what she could to conceive again. She was fortunate to conceive relatively quickly with clomid. This could have been from the combination of metformin and weight loss. Both weight loss and metformin use with or without clomid have been demonstrated to be effective in promoting pregnancy in women with PCOS. Originally, much of the nutrition session was spent educating her about PCOS and how insulin resistance plays such an important role. The importance of selecting whole grain carbohydrate sources over her high intake of refined foods and eating often were the primary focus. Teresa was able to see the benefits of this as she experienced reduced cravings for sweets and hypoglycemic episodes.

Once Teresa became pregnant, the focus shifted to helping her eat a diet that would best support her pregnancy, avoid miscarriage and obstetrical complications such as GDM. Although it was not diagnosed, I treated Teresa as if it was already known that she had GDM. Nutrition recommendations included emphasis on consuming moderate amounts of whole grains, limiting refined foods and sweetened beverages, eating often, distributing carbohydrates evenly throughout the day and having protein-rich foods at all meals and snacks.

Future follow-up sessions would enable the dietitian to assess Teresa's diet for nutritional adequacy and proper weight gain. It would also provide an opportunity for the dietitian to discuss the many benefits of breastfeeding for her and for her baby. The importance of self-care after her baby is born including eating and exercise strategies could also be explored. In addition, motivational interviewing could be used to potentially increase her motivation to increase her physical activity.

CASE 2

Jamie was a 16 year-old who originally came to see me in April for nutrition counseling for weight loss. For most of her life, Jamie struggled with her weight. At age 8 she tried her first diet, Weight Watchers, in which she had limited success. Last summer, Jamie went to a weight loss camp for 2 months and lost 9 pounds; she was not able to maintain it and regained it all. She has been on and off various other diets for the past year with limited success.

Jamie's parents were very concerned about her weight which was increasing. They were finding junk food hidden in her room and candy wrappers in her backpack. Both parents were slender and very health conscious. They did not buy junk food and said they ate a low carbohydrate diet. Jamie was adopted and had a body type different from her parents. She was an only child. From the start, it was clear that Jamie was angry with her parents for trying to manage her food intake and that many battles had been fought over the dinner table. Although she was reluctant to see a nutritionist, Jamie admitted she was unhappy with the excess weight in her mid-section as she had a hard time finding clothes that fit, especially the kind that her friends wore. She also hated her stretch marks on her stomach and desired a thinner face.

Jamie was 5'4" and weighed 225 pounds. At the time of our visit this was her highest weight. Three months ago at her doctors she weighed 208 pounds. Most of Jamie's weight was centered in her abdominal area.

Jamie said she was depressed and had been seeing a therapist for the past year and a half. She was not on any medications for her depression. Socially, Jamie had a boyfriend who went to a different school but few close friends. She was a singer and really enjoyed music.

I met with Jamie alone for the first part of the nutrition assessment. When I probed about eating disorder behaviors, Jamie admitted to bingeing about once or twice a week on sweets. She also had a history of self-induced vomiting that started when she was in 8th grade. However, the last time she purged was in December. She denied any recent urges for this behavior. She also denied ever using laxatives, diuretics, or diet pills. Jamie belonged to a gym that she visited once a week.

Medically, Jamie reported having irregular periods. She saw a gynecologist recently who prescribed birth control medication to regulate her menstrual cycle. Jamie also reported feeling very tired and experiencing signs of hypoglycemia several times during the day. She said she had strong cravings for carbohydrate foods, saying "I just have to have it." She also admitted to difficulty recognizing when she was full as she could "eat and eat." Jamie had severe acne on her face and reported hair loss. Below is her 24-hour recall:

<u>24-hour food recall (without bingeing):</u>
Breakfast (6:50 a.m.): 16 oz. chocolate soy milk and granola or protein bar

Lunch (12:45 p.m.): roast beef sandwich on white bread, French fries with French salad dressing, candy bar and 16 oz. water

Snack (3 p.m.): salsa and chips and candy bar bought at vending machine and 12 oz. water

Dinner (6:30 p.m.): ½ cup butternut squash, ½ cup low-calorie apple sauce, 8 oz. grilled chicken and 12 oz. seltzer water

Nutrition analysis (using mypyramidtracker.gov): 2383 calories, 133 grams (22%) protein, 240 grams (42%) carbohydrate, 22 grams fiber, 102 grams (29%) fat, 30 grams (11%) saturated, 13 grams linoleic, 1 gram alpha-linolenic, 270 grams cholesterol, 580 mg calcium, 3,000 mg sodium.

Jamie's diet was high in saturated fat, sodium, and refined carbohydrates. Her fruit and vegetable intake was severely limited and her calcium intake was well below required amounts. There were 6 hours between her breakfast and lunch and her afternoon snack consisted of mainly carbohydrates.

I educated Jamie on the benefits of eating more frequently throughout the day with protein at all meals and snacks to decrease carbohydrate cravings and hypoglycemia. Together, we made a list of sample meals and snacks she could have at home and in the morning at school. The benefits of listening to internal cues of hunger and satiety were discussed. Jamie agreed to keep food records and "experiment" with rating her hunger and satisfaction levels with meals, recognizing which combination of foods would satisfy her the most. Finally, I encouraged Jamie to be more physically active.

The possibility of Jamie having PCOS was suspected due to the following: a history of irregular menses, weight gain in her mid-section, strong carbohydrate cravings and hypoglycemia, acne, and hair loss. All this was explained to Jamie and her mother. A referral was made to a reproductive endocrinologist who specializes in PCOS for further evaluation.

Jamie's goals:
1. Keep food records and record level of hunger and satisfaction with meals.
2. Eat every 3-5 hours with protein at all meals and snacks (especially morning and afternoon snacks).
3. Visit gym 3x/week for 40 minutes.
4. Schedule appointment with reproductive endocrinologist.
5. Follow-up visit for 2 weeks.

Follow-up session (2 weeks later)
Jamie said she was eating more often and trying to make sure to include protein with her meals. However, it was difficult eating protein with snacks at school. Together, we reviewed her food records from the past 2 weeks. Jamie attempted rating her degree of hunger and fullness but said she was having difficulty distinguishing when she was satisfied. She noticed the connection of having more protein and experiencing less hypoglycemia and cravings for sweets. Her food records revealed one day of bingeing after school on candy that she bought at a drugstore on her way home. She realized, while reviewing food records, that she did not eat enough protein with her lunch that day. Jamie went to the gym one day for 30 minutes.

At this session I educated Jamie on how food affects blood sugar levels and the differences between whole grain and refined carbohydrates. We also talked about the benefits of fruits and vegetables. Food models were used to show Jamie examples of serving sizes. We came up with a list of snacks Jamie could have at school that required no refrigeration. I also explored reasons why she binged and suggested things she could do to cope with intense feelings instead of using food for support. Since Jamie did not increase her exercise, we explored her resistance toward it. She said her mother was always bothering her to go to the gym. It was also revealed that she enjoyed dancing to music.

Jamie's goals:
1. Continue keeping food records, rating hunger and satiety levels.
2. Continue eating every 3-5 hours, especially morning snack at school.
3. Dancing to music in her room, 2 days per week for 30 minutes.
4. Apply two coping skills before bingeing.
5. Appointment scheduled next week with reproductive endocrinologist.

Second Followup Session (2 weeks later)
Jamie saw the reproductive endocrinologist who diagnosed her with PCOS. She was prescribed 2,000 mg of metformin daily which she started taking. Jamie complained that the pill size of metformin was "huge." She didn't report experiencing any side effects. The report sent from her physician indicated insulin resistance and hyperandrogenism.

Since we last met, Jamie was pleased to announce that she had not binged and even applied some of the coping skills we came up with when she had urges. She was able to add in a morning snack at school on some days but forgot on others. Jamie was still keeping food records and rating her hunger and satiety levels. She was able to do some dancing in her room and said she enjoyed it. Although I did not weigh Jamie, she reported her clothes fitting looser.

Food records show Jamie was eating more whole grain carbo- hydrates and less food overall. On some days there were still long periods of time between meals. Although she did add more fruit into her diet, they were still very limited as were vegetables.

With her parents present, I further explained what PCOS was and how her signs and symptoms are connected with it, especially elevated insulin levels and cravings for carbohydrates and weight gain. We discussed the nutrition recommendations for PCOS. We also discussed the importance of taking metformin daily with food and that it was not a substitute for healthy eating. I recommended Jamie supplement with vitamin D because of her low intake of vitamin D containing foods and because she was obese. I also recommended cinnamon extract and fish oil supplements regularly. The benefits of exercise were reiterated. Jamie said she could do more dancing at home to music. She also agreed to add in more fruits.

Jamie's goals:
1. Continue with goals set at last session (hunger satiety work, eating often, and applying coping skills).
2. Dancing to music in her room, 3-4 days per week for 30 minutes.
3. Increase fruits to 2 servings per day.
4. Take 3 grams of cinnamon extract, 1,000 IU of vitamin D, and 1-3 grams of fish oil supplements in addition to a multi-vitamin daily.
5. Follow-up visit for 2 weeks.

Although Jamie started nutrition counseling at her parent's request, she was able to acknowledge that she wanted to lose weight. The focus in the first sessions was aimed at developing a relationship with Jamie, and most of the nutrition assessment was spent without her mother present. In this way, she was able to open up and explore her feelings about food and weight. Screening questions in the nutrition assessment revealed a history of bingeing and purging behaviors. They also revealed the possibility of Jamie having PCOS due to her struggles with weight, the location of her weight in her mid-section, cravings for sweets and hypoglycemic episodes as well as irregular periods and hair loss. This enabled her to get properly tested by a physician who prescribed her with an insulin-sensitizer.

Because Jamie was a binge eater and had a long history of dieting, calories or a specific meal plan for weight loss were not discussed. Instead, I focused on helping her stabilize her eating patterns by trusting her body for food amounts, not bingeing or dieting. Since I highly suspected she had PCOS, I provided nutrition recommendations appropriate for the syndrome. Emphasis was placed on consuming whole grain carbohydrates rather than refined ones. Small obtainable goals, set together, were provided at each session. Through exploration, Jamie admitted being resistant to exercising at the gym because of pressure from her mother. Instead, we were able to come up with an activity she liked to do.

Communication with Jamie's therapist was essential as it was apparent Jamie was angry with her parent's control over her weight and was affecting her eating behaviors. Jamie's parents were educated on the benefits of the mindful eating approach I was supporting her with instead of a diet plan. Her family was educated about PCOS, and was very grateful that I suspected it so she could get proper treatment.

Future nutrition sessions would be needed to assess Jamie's compliance with her eating and exercise plan as well as medication use, since she was adverse to the large size of the pill. It would also provide opportunity to further explore attitudes about food and weight and reinforce mindful eating. Since Jamie's diet was high in saturated fat and limited in fruits and vegetables, further dietary goals that addressed this would be needed to prevent dyslipidemia. Also, it would be helpful for her physician to check her vitamin D levels and repeat blood work after 3 months. Improvements in her lab results could positively reinforce the changes Jamie made in her eating.

CASE 3

Elsa was a 32 year-old woman who was diagnosed with Polycystic Ovary Syndrome (PCOS) four years ago. She had a history of irregular menstrual periods, occurring every three to four months and lasting six days, on average. Her physical exam noted excess facial hair on the upper lip and the chest; lab results showed elevated androgen levels. In addition, Elsa had hypertension, dyslipidemia, and insulin resistance with hyperinsulinemia (her clinical profile is shown in Table 1). Elsa was single, worked full time in a government office job and lived with and cared for her grandmother. She was inactive, but had a gym membership and stated that she liked to dance.

Elsa's doctor had prescribed blood pressure medicine last year, but she had resisted taking it. She had been on 2,000 mg/day of metformin, although she confessed that she was "sporadic" in taking her medications as she 'hated' taking pills. Metformin is an insulin sensitizing drug that has been shown to have positive effects on lipid profiles in women with PCOS. She had also been prescribed Lovaza™, an omega-3 polyunsaturated fatty-acid derived medication for high triglycerides.

Elsa was referred for nutrition counseling by her doctor due to the symptoms of PCOS, dyslipidemia and hypertension. She had a positive family history for diabetes and hypertension. Her mother had diabetes and she "didn't want to prick her fingers like her mom did." Elsa was 5'6" and weighed 253 pounds, which was her highest weight to date. Based on her BMI of 41 and a waist circumference of 57 inches, she was morbidly obese. However, she admitted her motivation for the consult was not weight loss. She had been heavy since childhood, but she was motivated to reduce her risk for developing diabetes and she wanted to stop taking medications.

Table 1. Clinical Profile for Elsa

Lab Test	Results	Normal Ranges	Significance
Blood pressure	142 / 91	<140/90 mm/Hg	Borderline High
Insulin (fasting)	18.4	<10 mIU/L	↑ insulin resistance
TSH	0.63	.40 – 5.50 uIU/mL	WNL
Testosterone	68	20-75 mg/dL (ideal <50)	WNL (therapeutic goal <50 mg/dl)
HbA1C	6.1	<6.0%	↑ impaired glucose tolerance, pre-diabetes
Glucose (fasting)	110	70 – 126 mg/dL	↑ impaired glucose tolerance, pre-diabetes
Total Cholesterol	263	<200 mg/dL	↑ hypercholesterolemia
LDL Cholesterol	183	<100 mg/dL	↑ hypercholesterolemia
Triglycerides	630	<150 mg/dl	↑ hypertriglyceridemia

Nutrition Assessment

During the initial nutrition assessment, Elsa stated that she had limited cooking skills, relied on convenience and fast foods during the day and prepared only the evening meal at home. A 24-hour dietary recall that mirrored her typical diet showed the following:

Breakfast (8:30 am): a soft pretzel with mustard or a bagel or muffin with butter

Morning Snack (10:00 am): crackers, trail mix or a candy bar

Lunch (12:30 pm): purchased at a work food cart or fast food restaurant and consisted of a hamburger or meatball sandwich, large soda (16 oz), a bag of chips or a side of soup (chicken noodle)

Afternoon snack (2:30 pm): cup of tea with regular sugar as she did not like sugar substitutes

Dinner (5:30 pm.): some type of beef, a salad and two biscuits

Evening snack (8:00 pm): lightly salted peanuts and/or pretzels

In addition, Elsa reported that she did not drink alcohol, but she consumed 64 oz. of fruit juice every day, drinking approximately 24 oz. at breakfast, 24 oz. for lunch and through the afternoon and 12 oz. at dinner. She also reported intense carbohydrate cravings.

A diet analysis was done of her 24-hour recall using a computerized diet analysis program (www.NutriBase.com). Elsa ate 147% of recommended calories (3,236 calories/day), with 12% (97g) of total calories from protein, 62% (501g) from carbohydrate, and only eight grams of fiber (32% of recommended). The percentage of total calories from fat was 27% (97g) with over three times (32%) the recommended amount for saturated fat. Cholesterol intake was within a recommended amount (242 mg) but her sodium intake was 5,132 mg, which was 223% over the recommended amount of 2,300 mg.

Elsa's diet was high in total calories, saturated fats, sodium and refined carbohydrates. She was void of antioxidant, fiber-rich fruits, vegetables and calcium food sources such as dairy. She ate more fruits and vegetables during the summer months but during the winter months, rarely ate fresh fruit. She did occasionally have a fruit cup at work. Most of her carbohydrate intake was from simple sugars, in large part due to the consumption of fruit juice and soda. She stated that giving up the fruit juice would be a difficult thing for her to do. The intake of convenience and fast foods were responsible for the excessive sodium and saturated fats found in her diet. Elsa denied the use of any eating disorder behaviors including binge eating but did admit to eating at times when she wasn't hungry.

The dietitian and Elsa reviewed how insulin resistance and excess body weight contributed to PCOS and an increased the risk for diabetes. She explained how diet and exercise could reduce these risk factors. The dietitian also encouraged Elsa to take her prescribed medications; metformin, Lovaza™ and her blood pressure medicine on a regular basis to benefit her in regulating her glucose and insulin levels, weight loss, dyslipidemia and her blood pressure.

Nutrition education during the first session focused on how food affects blood sugar and how protein and fiber in her meals and snacks can mediate blood sugar and insulin levels. Food sources of proteins were discussed and Elsa was given a handout of low-fat and plant-based proteins. Whole grains versus refined grains were defined. Together, they worked on how to replace the refined grains in Elsa's diet with whole grains. Also, she was used to drinking 64 oz. of fruit juice daily and stated her resistance to changing this habit. Motivational interviewing was used to encourage Elsa to decrease her intake of juice and reduce the calories and simple sugars in her diet. Elsa spaced her meals and snacks throughout the day but many of her food choices were high in saturated fat and refined sugars, and low in protein. Elsa was enthusiastic in making dietary changes to improve her PCOS symptoms and reduce her risk for diabetes.

Based on her dietary analysis and diagnosis, dietary and lifestyle goals for Elsa should include a meal plan that supports a reduced calorie intake and increase in physical activity with a goal of 7 – 10% reduction in body weight. The diet should include an increase in dietary protein to decrease carbohydrate cravings, plus more unsaturated fats and dietary fiber to promote satiety and improve dyslipidemia. Carbohydrates should be reduced to a moderate level. Refined or simple carbohydrates should be replaced with whole grains and carbohydrate intake should be spread evenly throughout the day. For the initial appointment, Elsa's nutrition goals included:

1. Continue to eat 5-6 times throughout the day.
2. Incorporate lean protein-rich sources at each meal and snack.
3. Replace refined grains with whole grains.
4. Limit the amount of fruit juice in her diet to 3 servings per day.
5. Increase whole fruit consumption to one per day.

Follow-up Session

Elsa returned for a three week follow-up appointment. She had successfully decreased the amount of fruit juice she consumed but had not added fruit. Her diet was still low in fiber. She had tried to include low-fat proteins in her diet but stated it was difficult as she ate both breakfast and lunch away from home. The dietitian and Elsa worked on building meal plans from the restaurant and food cart for her lunches that were lower in calories with low-fat protein and reduced sodium. Elsa felt the meal plans would benefit her in making healthier food choices. She also agreed to eat breakfast at home as well as take a morning and afternoon snack with protein with her to work. Breakfast meal plans included oatmeal with milk, cottage cheese and fruit and one egg with whole wheat toast. Snack suggestions included fruit, trail mix, yogurt and nuts. She was still inactive but stated she was interested in starting a dance class. Her nutrition goals for the second appointment included:

1. Continue decreasing the amount of fruit juice in diet through dilution or replacement of juice with a non-caloric beverage.
2. Increase consumption of whole grains.
3. Work on having a low calorie, low-fat, low sodium lunch at least 2 times per week from the food cart or fast food restaurant.
4. Eat breakfast at home and bring at least two snacks to work.

Second follow-up session

One month later, Elsa came to her second follow-up appointment. She reported having a difficult time reducing the fruit juice and was still consuming 64 ounces per day. However, she had added a piece of fruit each day, usually an orange in mid-morning. She increased her consumption of vegetables in the evening meal and made an effort to eat whole grain bread. She was consistent in eating breakfast at home three times per week, but other days ate a bagel or pretzel from the food cart at work. On most days she brought at least one snack with her to work. She reported not eating an afternoon snack and was still not active. She had not lost any weight.

For this session, the dietitian used food models and the plate method to educate Elsa on portion control. Attention to hunger and fullness cues were discussed and the importance of reducing simple carbohydrates was stressed. Together, they discussed alternative beverages and strategies such as drinking water or diet drinks to reduce fruit juice consumption. She was also going a long time between meals, especially from lunch until dinner. Snacks that contained some protein were reviewed, including nuts that could be purchased from the food cart at her work. Since Elsa said she liked dancing and belonged to a gym, the role of physical activity to improve insulin resistance and promote weight loss was discussed. Taking dance classes offered at her gym was encouraged and Elsa agreed to sign up for the classes. The nutrition goals for Elsa centered around learning to be mindful of hunger and satiety cues and portion control. She was encouraged to keep food records and write down how hungry and/or satisfied she felt prior to and after eating. They discussed the importance of protein at each meal and snack in order to promote satiety and eating often throughout the day.

Third follow-up session

Elsa returned in 1 month for her appointment. She saw her physician the day before and was happy to report that she had lost 5 pounds. Repeat blood work showed slight reductions in fasting insulin, total cholesterol, and LDL levels. Her triglyceride levels were 430 mg/dl and blood pressure was 130/82, both significant reductions. A review of her dietary intake showed that she returned to drinking the fruit juice, but was not drinking it at dinner and she did not miss it like she thought she would. She agreed to continue to work at reducing the fruit juice in her diet. Portion sizes had been reduced and Elsa was eating some protein with all of her meals and snacks. She stated she was not feeling as hungry or having the carbohydrates cravings. The dietitian reviewed food records with Elsa that showed she was practicing listening to internal cues of hunger and fullness. Her overall caloric intake was reduced. She had been eating breakfast at home almost every day using the meal plans she created with the dietitian and she added a fruit cup to her afternoon snack. Elsa attended two ballroom dance classes and was enjoying them. She also stated she was now taking metformin daily and her menstrual periods had become more regular.

Elsa announced she had accepted a job out of town and this would be her last appointment. Elsa had come to the dietitian wanting to reduce the risk of diabetes and to stop taking her medications. Through intensive, personalized nutrition education and monitoring her dietary and lifestyle changes at follow-up appointments, the dietitian assisted Elsa in making the changes in her diet to promote weight loss, improve insulin resistance, dyslipidemia, and blood pressure. Continued follow-up sessions would have allowed the dietitian to work with Elsa on specific dietary goals that would benefit her such as the Dietary Approach to Stop Hypertension (DASH) diet for hypertension or using the Glycemic Index as a strategy to reduce the insulin response to carbohydrates in the body. The dietitian finished up the session with a summary of Elsa's dietary and lifestyle goals and presented her with referral phone numbers for a medical team in her new town, including a registered dietitian who worked with women with PCOS in order to provide a seamless transition of care.

All of these case studies demonstrate the importance of medical nutrition therapy in the treatment of women with PCOS. Adequate knowledge and training, along with a high degree of suspicion, can allow dietetic professionals to identify patients who may have PCOS and recommend further diagnostic testing. Since women with PCOS are at a higher risk for developing chronic disease, mood disorders, and infertility, education on diet and lifestyle modification are imperative. Thus, dietitians play an important role in the recognition, prevention, and treatment of PCOS.

APPENDIX 1.
SAMPLE MENU PLANS FOR POLYCYSTIC OVARY SYNDROME

1200-1400 Calorie Sample Menu / Polycystic Ovary Syndrome

<u>**Breakfast**</u>
1 Fruit
1-2 Proteins
1-2 Breads/Starches
1 Fat

<u>Example</u>
1 cup melon
1 cup soy milk, nonfat
¾ cup oatmeal, cooked
1 T almonds

<u>**Lunch**</u>
1-2 Breads/Starches
3 Proteins
2-3 Vegetables

1 Fruit
2 Fats

1 whole grain roll
7 ½ oz. tofu
2 cups spinach salad with
assorted vegetables
orange
4 walnuts
1 T Vinaigrette dressing

<u>**Snack**</u>
1-2 Fats
1 Protein
1 Fruit

1 T peanut butter
apple

<u>**Dinner**</u>
3-5 Proteins

2 Vegetables

1-2 Fats
1-2 Breads/Starches

4 oz. skinless chicken
1 oz. low-fat feta cheese
1 cup green beans and
1 cup salad
1 T Italian dressing
¾ cup brown rice

23% protein, 40% carbohydrate, 37% fat, 6% saturated fat, 13.5% MUFA, 14% PUFA, 144 g cholesterol, 31g fiber, 850 mg calcium, 2,100 mg sodium

1500-1700 Calorie Sample Menu / Polycystic Ovary Syndrome

<u>Breakfast</u>   <u>Example</u>
1 Fruit   1 cup grapes
1-2 Protein   ½ cup low-fat cottage cheese
1-2 Breads/Starches   2 slices whole grain toast
1-2 Fats   1 T of peanut butter

<u>Snack</u>
1 Protein   1 oz. low-fat cheese
1 Bread/Starch   6 whole wheat crackers

<u>Lunch</u>
2-3 Vegetables   1 ½ cups romaine lettuce
                                     and assorted vegetables
3 Proteins   4 oz. grilled chicken
2 Fats   2 T lite caesar salad dressing
2 Breads/Starches   1 cup low-sodium
                                     minestrone soup
                                     ¼ cup croutons

<u>Snack</u>
1 Protein   1/3 cup edamame
1 Fruit   pear

<u>Dinner</u>
4-6 Proteins   4 oz. salmon
2 Vegetables   1 cup broccoli
1-2 Fats   1 tsp olive oil
1-2 Breads/Starches   ½ cup sweet potatoes

<u>Snack</u>
1 Fat   ¼ cup almonds
1 Fruit   plum

24% protein, 44% carbohydrate, 35 g fiber, 34% fat, 5% saturated, 16% MUFA, 9% PUFA, 155 mg cholesterol, 920 mg calcium, 2,300 mg sodium

1800-2000 Calorie Sample Menu / Polycystic Ovary Syndrome

Breakfast   **Example**
1-2 Breads/Starches   ½ cup quinoa, cooked
1 Fruit   ¾ cup blueberries
1-2 Proteins   ¾ cup soymilk, nonfat
1-2 Fats   1 T almonds

Mid-Morning Snack   **Example**
1 Protein   1 cup soymilk, nonfat
1 Fruit   1 small banana

Lunch   **Example**
1-2 Breads/Starches   1 whole wheat bun
3 Proteins   1 veggie burger with 1 oz. low-fat
cheese
2-3 Vegetables   1 cup mixed greens
1 Fruit   1 apple
1-2 Fat   s 1 T Italian dressing

Mid Afternoon Snack   **Example**
1 Protein   4 oz. plain yogurt, low-fat
1 Fruit   1 peach
1 Fat   1 T flaxseed

Dinner   **Example**
2 Breads/Starches   ¾ cup bulgur pilaf
4 Proteins   5 oz. pork tenderloin
2-3 Vegetables   1 cup mixed vegetables, steamed
1-2 Fats   1 tsp. olive oil

24% protein, 45% carbohydrate, 47 g fiber, 31% fat, 5% saturated, 11% MUFA, 10% PUFA, 823 mg calcium, 2,000 mg sodium

2000-2200 Calorie Sample Menu / Polycystic Ovary Syndrome

Breakfast   Example
1 Fruit   1 cup raspberries
1-2 Proteins   1 cup soy milk, nonfat
1-2 Breads/Starches   ½ cup homemade granola
                                 with oats
1-2 Fats   1 T flax seed

Snack
1 Protein   6 oz. plain yogurt, nonfat
1 Fruit   1 cup blueberries

Lunch
3 Proteins   1 oz. low-fat cheese
                                 2 egg omelet
1-2 Breads/Starches   2 slices whole wheat bread
2-3 Vegetables   1 cup mixed onions and peppers
1 Fruit   1 cup strawberries

Snack
1-2 Fat   8 walnuts
1 Fruit   1 cup pineapple
1 Breads/Starches   1 whole grain granola bar

Dinner
4-6 Proteins   6 oz. halibut, grilled
2 Vegetables   1 cup green beans, cooked
1-2 Fats   1 tsp olive oil and 1 T almonds
1-2 Breads/Starches   1 cup wild rice, cooked

20% protein, 36% carbohydrate, 43 g fiber, 44% fat, 7% saturated, 15% MUFA, 18% PUFA, 500 mg cholesterol, 900 mg calcium, 1,936 mg sodium

APPENDIX 2. RESOURCES FOR POLYCYSTIC OVARY SYNDROME

Consumer Education, Advocacy and Support Organizations

Children's Hospital of Boston
Center for Young Women's Health
www.youngwomenshealth.org/pcosinfo.html

Focuses on PCOS information for teenagers. This site has a great explanation of many common PCOS questions, featuring figures and graphs. It also includes information on reading food labels, recipes, snack ideas, sample menus, and worksheets for menu planning and exercise, all specifically for the PCOS teen.

OBGYN.net
www.obgyn.net

A good site for professionals and consumers to download. Includes professional publications about PCOS, including infertility, endometriosis, and hirsutism.

PCOS Nutrition
www.PCOSnutrition.com
(484) 252-9028

The personal website for Angela Grassi, MS, RD, LDN author of *The Dietitian's Guide to Polycystic Ovary Syndrome*. Provides nutrition and medical information for PCOS. Sign up for free monthly PCOS Nutrition Tips. Offers nutrition counseling by phone or in person for individuals with PCOS and eating disorders.

Polycystic Ovary Association
www.PCOSupport.org

The Polycystic Ovary Association website includes a member database to find professionals who treat PCOS. It also has research articles and provides chat rooms for different PCOS concerns (i.e. eating disorders, infertility, etc). The association hosts an annual conference for consumers.

Polycystic Ovary Syndrome of Australia
www.posaa.asn.au
Very similar to the Polycystic Ovary Association in the United States. This site also contains support, information, and advocacy for women with PCOS. The Australia website also includes chat rooms, message boards, professional database and annual conference.

Verity
www.verity-pcos.org.uk
Verity is the support organization for women with PCOS living in the United Kingdom. Use this site to find information and professionals. It has a newsletter, discussion board, and fact sheets. This organization also has an annual conference.

PCOS UK
www.pcos-uk.org.uk
PCOS UK is a multidisciplinary society for healthcare professionals caring for women with Polycystic Ovary Syndrome. It provides educational support to improve the awareness and knowledge of PCOS and related conditions among healthcare professionals in the UK.

Project PCOS
www.projectPCOS.org
Established by Ashley Tabeling, a woman with PCOS, this site provides awareness, information and support for women with PCOS from the top experts in the field. Find articles, recipes, learn how to be an advocate, and read personal stories. It is a great site to find PCOS treatment professionals and groups across the country.

PCOS Pals
www.health.groups.yahoo.com/group/PCOS-Pals/
On-line Yahoo message board where women can post questions and answers to common PCOS topics.

PCOS Today Magazine
www.PCOStodaymagazine.com
An e-zine dedicated to providing up to date information on PCOS including causes and treatment, resources, personal stories, book reviews and clinical trials.

Soulcysters
www.soulcysters.com
A great resource for women with PCOS. This website provides a good overview of symptoms, treatment, and other PCOS links. Also provides a message board where individuals can post questions and read others responses.
Professional Associations

Academy for Eating Disorders
www.aedweb.org
The Academy for Eating Disorders is an international professional organization that promotes excellence in research, treatment and prevention of eating disorders. The AED provides education, training and a forum for collaboration and professional dialogue. Use this site for links to professional publications on eating disorders and to locate a treatment professional. The AED hosts annual conference for professionals and local events.

American Dietetic Association
www.eatright.org
(800) 877-1600
The American Dietetic Association is the nation's largest organization for food and nutrition professionals. Use this site to find a registered dietitian, shop for books and gifts and search for food and nutrition information and publications. The ADA also hosts annual conference for professionals.

American Association of Clinical Endocrinologists

www.aace.com

A great site to find an endocrinologist in your area. The website provides advocacy, research articles, and information on upcoming meetings and events.

American College of Obstetricians and Gynecologists (ACOG)

www.acog.org

This site provides information on all aspects of women's health. Information pamphlets on PCOS available for purchase. This site can also be used to locate an OBGYN.

American Diabetes Association (ADA)

www.diabetes.org

A great resource for information on PCOS, insulin resistance, and diabetes. This site provides a research database with current clinical trials. A nutrition section provides information, recipes, tips on eating out and making healthy food choices.

American Heart Association

www.americanheart.org

The site for heart health. Find information fact sheets and tips on treating and preventing heart disease, diabetes, stroke, and hypertension. Professional publications and clinical updates are available. Use this site to find recipes, articles, nutrition tips for adults and children.

American Psychological Association (APA)

www.apa.org

Use this site to find a psychologist and obtain resources and information on treating emotional problems.

American Society for Reproductive Medicine
www.asrm.org
The ASRM is a multidisciplinary organization committed to the advancement of reproductive medicine by serving as the leading advocate for patient care, research and education. ASRM has information on infertility for professionals and consumers. Use the website to find a doctor, request information booklets, and links to adoption agencies.

National Eating Disorders Association
www.edap.org
A great resource that provides information and advocacy for eating disorders. Use this site to locate a treatment professional or download reproducible fact sheets and client handouts. This organization hosts an annual conference for consumers and professionals.

RESOLVE: The National Infertility Association
www.resolve.org
RESOLVE: The National Infertility Association, established in 1974, is a non-profit organization to promote reproductive health and to ensure equal access to all family building options for men and women experiencing infertility or other reproductive disorders. Resolve provides awareness, support and information to people who are experiencing infertility.

ALTERNATIVE AND COMPLEMENTARY MEDICINE RESOURCES

The Natural Medicines Comprehensive Database
www.NaturalDatabase.com
The largest and most detailed listing of non-biased natural medicines available. This database is a great place to look up information on supplements, including specific manufacturer brands. Membership is required to access the database.

National Center for Complementary and Alternative Medicine
www.nccam.nih.gov
Sponsored by the National Institute of Health, this federally funded site provides information on complementary and alternative medicine. This is another great place to look up information on supplements.

TRAINING RESOURCES FOR NUTRITION PROFESSIONALS

Molly Kellogg, RD, LCSW
www.mollykellogg.com
Molly is a therapist and a dietitian who provides resources for counseling excellence for nutrition professionals. Access her site to sign up for her free newsletter with counseling tips and to purchase her book, *Counseling Tips for Nutrition Therapists: Practice Workbook*, 2006. Molly also offers practical, hands-on training workshops, home study courses, and supervision by phone.

Understanding Nutrition
www.understandingnutrition.com
Jessica Setnick, MS, RD, LD provides training resources for professionals working with eating disorder clients. Sign up to attend Eating Disorder Boot Camp™ or purchase the home study version. Other resources available to health professionals including *The Eating Disorders Clinical Pocket Guide: Quick Reference for Health Care Providers*.

APPENDIX 3. COMMON IDC-9 CODES FOR PCOS AND RELATED CONDITIONS.

IDC-9 Code	Diagnosis:
706.10	Acne
704.00	Alopecia
626.00	Amenorrhea
307.10	Anorexia Nervosa
307.51	Bulimia Nervosa
250.00	Diabetes Type 2
307.50	Eating Disorder Not Otherwise Specified
648.83	Gestational Diabetes Mellitus
642.33	Gestational Hypertension
271.90	Glucose Intolerance
704.10	Hirsutism
272.00	Hypercholesterolemia
401.10	Hypertension
790.60	Hyperglycemia (without diabetes)
272.20	Hyperlipidemia, mixed
251.10	Hyperinsulinemia
272.10	Hypertriglyceridemia
251.20	Hypoglycemia, unspecified, nondiabetic
244.90	Hypothyroid
628.90	Infertility, unspecified
564.10	Irritable Bowel Syndrome
277.70	Metabolic Syndrome
278.00	Obesity, NOS
733.90	Osteopenia
733.00	Osteoporosis
278.02	Overweight
256.40	Polycystic Ovarian Syndrome
642.40	Pre-eclampsia
327.23	Sleep Apnea

INDEX